Holger Pettersson · Dempsey S. Springfield
William F. Enneking

Radiologic
Management of
Musculoskeletal
Tumors

With 112 Figures

Springer-Verlag
London Berlin Heidelberg New York
Paris Tokyo

Holger Pettersson, MD
Visiting Professor, Department of Radiology, University of Florida
College of Medicine, Gainesville, Florida, USA
Associate Professor, Chief of Section for Skeletal Radiology, and
Chairman, Department of Radiology, University of Lund, Sweden

Dempsey S. Springfield, MD
Associate Professor and Chief of Orthopedic Oncology, Department
of Orthopedics, University of Florida College of Medicine, Gainesville,
Florida, USA

William F. Enneking, MD
Distinguished Service Professor and Eugene L. Jewett Professor of
Orthopedic Surgery, Department of Orthopedics, University of
Florida College of Medicine, Gainesville, Florida, USA

Contributing author

Irvin F. Hawkins, Jr., MD
Professor of Radiology and Surgery and Chief of Interventional
Radiology, Department of Radiology, University of Florida College
of Medicine, Gainesville, Florida, USA

ISBN-13: 978-1-4471-1420-8   e-ISBN: 978-1-4471-1418-5

DOI: 10.1007/978-1-4471-1418-5

Library of Congress Cataloging-in-Publication Data
Pettersson, Holger, 1942–
Radiologic staging in muscoloskeletal tumors.
Includes bibliographies and index.
1. Musculoskeletal system—Tumors—Diagnosis. 2. Musculoskeletal system—
Radiography. 3. Diagnostic imaging. I. Springfield, Dempsey S., 1945–
II. Enneking, William F., 1926– . III. Title.
DNLM: 1. Bone Neoplasms—radiography. 2. Musculoskeletal System—radiography.
3. Neoplasm Staging. WE 141 P499r
ISBN-13: 978-1-4471-1420-8

© Springer-Verlag Berlin Heidelberg 1987
Softcover reprint of the hardcover 1st Edition 1987

The use of registered names, trademarks, etc. in this publication does not imply, even
in the absence of a specific statement, that such names are exempt from the relevant
protective laws and regulations and therefore free for general use.

Product Liability: The publisher can give no guarantee for information about drug
dosage and application thereof contained in this book. In every individual case the
respective user must check its accuracy by consulting other pharmaceutical literature.

Filmset and printed by BAS Printers Limited, Over Wallop, Hampshire
2128/3916 543210

Preface

During the last decade the therapeutic approach to musculoskeletal tumors has changed dramatically, from ablative surgery with amputation of the limb to reconstructive surgery with transplantation of bone and vessels combined with radio- and chemotherapy. This has changed the demands on radiologists and pathologists to a considerable degree. At the same time there has been a manifold increase in the diagnostic possibilities offered by modern radiology, with several new modalities affording a potential for morphologic depiction and tissue characterization that was unattainable a decade ago.

Today, the definitive diagnostic work-up and treatment of patients with musculoskeletal tumors is most often done in tumor centers, by groups that ideally should be composed of an orthopedic surgeon, radiotherapist, oncologist, radiologist, pathologist and cytologist. It is necessary for all the members of this team to be well versed in the surgical and other treatment principles, in the pathologic concepts, and in the radiologic interpretation of musculoskeletal tumors. Moreover, it is important that the modern diagnostic approach to musculoskeletal tumors is well known also at the referring center, be it a private practitioner's office or a large hospital. This will avoid unnecessary biopsies, and repetition of radiologic and other diagnostic procedures that have already been performed at the referring center.

The present book is written by two orthopedic surgeons and a radiologist at the University of Florida College of Medicine, Gainesville, Florida, which is one of the largest musculoskeletal tumor centers in the United States. Based on modern pathologic and surgical principles, the book is intended as a concise discussion of modern radiologic approaches to the preoperative work-up of musculoskeletal tumors. It is the authors' hope that the book will serve as a source of knowledge and understanding of how musculoskeletal tumors should be managed radiologically. It is not meant solely for the members of the treatment teams in tumor centers, but also for all those referring orthopedic surgeons and radiologists who only seldom see such patients.

Gainesville, Florida
September 1986

Holger Pettersson
Dempsey S. Springfield
William F. Enneking

Acknowledgments

We want to express our sincere gratitude and appreciation to the following institutions and people:

Technicare Corporation, USA and Europe, and TA Bioteknik AB, Sweden, for valuable economic support;

The NIH for financial support from grants NIH CA 16559 and NIH P 41RR02278, and the Medical Research Service of the Veterans Administration for financial help also;

John Davis for talented editorial assistance with the manuscript;

Our colleagues at the Department of Radiology, Orthopedic Surgery and Pathology, for advice and professional contributions;

And especially, Suzanne S. Spanier, MD, for her devoted work and her invaluable commitment to exploring the exciting and intriguing correlation of clinical, radiologic, and pathologic findings.

Contents

Chapter 1
General Pathologic Principles of Musculoskeletal Neoplasia

The terms "neoplasia" and "neoplasm" are difficult to define accurately. Robbins and Cotram (1979a) suggest that "a neoplasia is a new growth, comprising an abnormal collection of cells the growth of which exceeds and is uncoordinated with that of the normal tissue." This is a broad definition and in the musculoskeletal system there are neoplasms that grow in this uncoordinated way for a while but subsequently heal and are spontaneously converted to the appropriate normal tissue (e.g. non-ossifying fibroma). There are also neoplasms that will destroy all normal structures they encounter and disseminate throughout the patient causing death (e.g. Ewing's sarcoma). These are the two extremes and between them there is a broad spectrum of neoplasms.

Pathologists divide neoplastic tumors into two major groups: those that can metastasize (malignant) and those that cannot (benign). Experience has taught the histologic clues which indicate whether or not a specific tumor has the ability to invade local lymph or capillary channels and grow in a distant site. These clues include the number of mitoses per high-power magnification field, the presence of abnormal mitoses, nuclear and cellular morphology, necrosis, and vascular invasion (Enzinger and Weiss 1983). There are other histologic indicators which suggest whether the tumor is a locally aggressive, rapidly growing lesion or a more indolent process, but the clinical course and radiologic presentation are often more accurate in classifying the local behavior of tumors.

Growth Patterns

The growth patterns of benign neoplasms can be classified according to the relationship of the tumor to its capsule. Those *benign tumors* which grow without invading the surrounding tissue and are truly encapsulated constitute one category. These lesions are the least aggressive tumors, usually grow slowly and often heal spontaneously. Some tumors in this category require surgical removal, but surgery can be quite limited and local recurrence is rare.

The other major category of benign tumors consists of lesions that invade the surrounding tissue and in which the apparent capsule (the pseudocapsule) is actually infiltrated by tumor cells. These tumors usually grow more rapidly than the non-invasive benign tumors and do not heal spontaneously. The margin of the surgical incision should be beyond the pseudocapsule. Within this category there is quite a variation in the degree of infiltration, from very limited infiltration of the pseudocapsule to very aggressive penetration. Usually the degree of invasiveness is indicated by the appropriate diagnostic studies.

Malignant tumors can be divided into two major treatment categories on the basis of their growth pattern and histologic presentation. The less aggressive type has a local growth pattern that is similar to that of the more aggressive benign tumors. These low-grade tumors are surrounded by reactive tissue and compress structures displaced by their growth. This reactive tissue forms a pseudocapsule which is invaded by nodules of neoplastic cells know as "satellites" (Fig. 1.1). As the tumor grows it resorbs the surrounding normal tissue through enzymic degradation. Low-grade lesions usually grow slowly, are associated with minimal symptoms and rarely metastasize. Their histologic grade in Broder's system is usually 1 or 2 (Robbins and Cotran 1979b).

The more aggressive malignant tumors invade the pseudocapsule and usually extend beyond it into the surrounding normal tissue. They grow rapidly, usually infiltrate the surrounding tissue before resorbing it, and elicit a modest reactive inflammatory response. Their metastatic rate is high and their histologic grade in Broder's system is usually 3 or 4. Nodules of tumor which are outside the reactive rim are called "skip lesions".

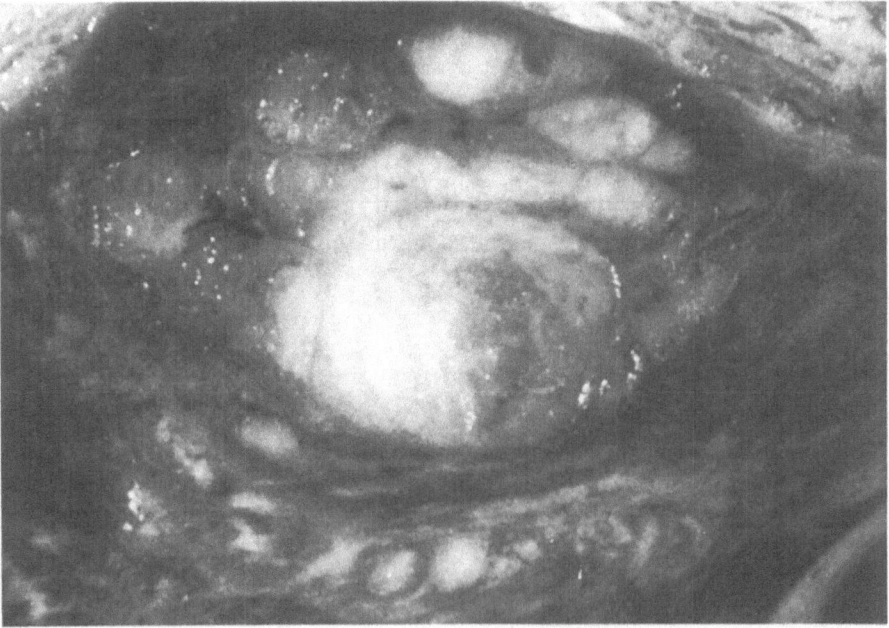

Fig. 1.1. Specimen of soft tissue sarcoma with "satellites." The numerous small nodules in the reactive tissue around the tumor are macroscopic satellites. Microscopic satellite nodules are also present.

Pathways of Growth

Musculoskeletal tumors grow along pathways of least resistance, directed by natural barriers. The cortex of bone is a modest barrier and is penetrated by tumors quite easily, while the periosteum is not so easily breached and often contains an aggressive benign tumor or one of low-grade malignancy. The medullary canal offers no restriction to growth and a primary bone tumor usually extends further intraosseously than it does extraosseously (Fig. 1.2). Cartilage, both epiphyseal and articular, is a very effective barrier which is only rarely penetrated. However, as the epiphysis begins to close and vascular channels cross the epiphyseal plate, the tumor may stream through these channels. Articular cartilage is rarely violated, and although giant cell tumor can penetrate cartilage, most primary bone tumors that invade an adjacent joint do so by escaping the bone at the ligamentous or synovial attachments (Fig. 1.3). In soft tissue the muscle fascia provides a minimal

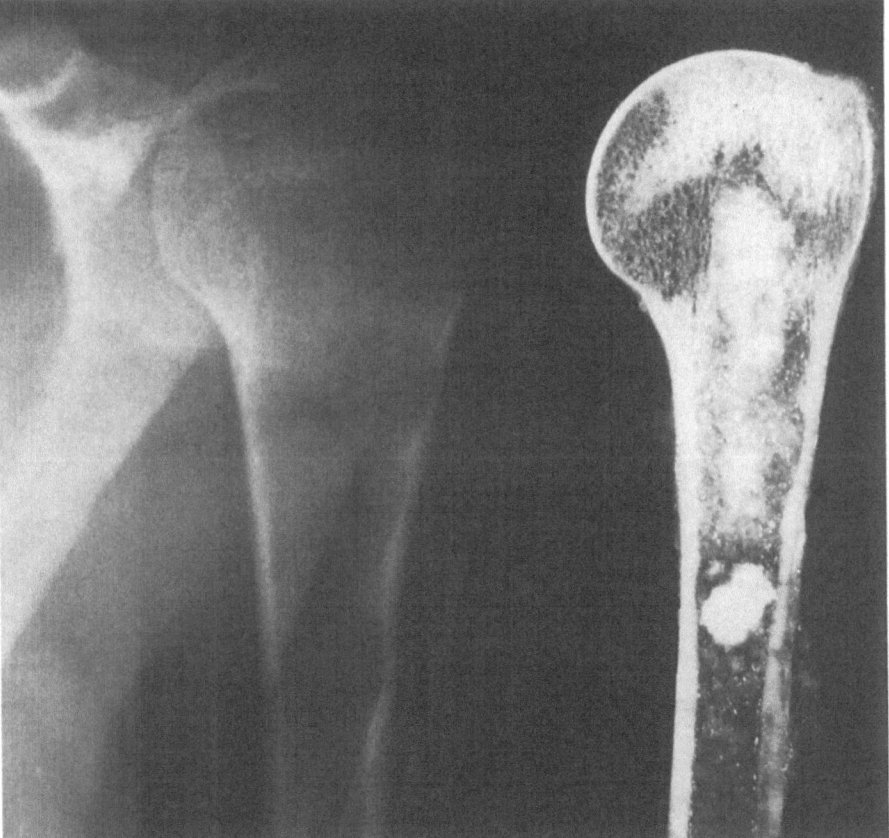

Fig. 1.2. Low-grade intraosseous chondrosarcoma: plain radiography and specimen. The tumor has eroded the endosteal surface of the bone but has not penetrated the cortex. Note that the longitudinal extension is greater than the circumferential extension.

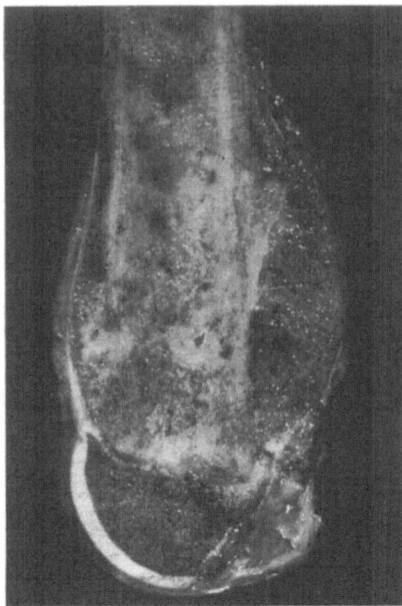

Fig. 1.3. Osteosarcoma of the distal femur: specimen. The periosteum is raised and penetrated. There has been extension into the joint via the posterior cruciate ligament. Note that the epiphyseal plate has slowed the tumor extension but has been penetrated in the posterior half.

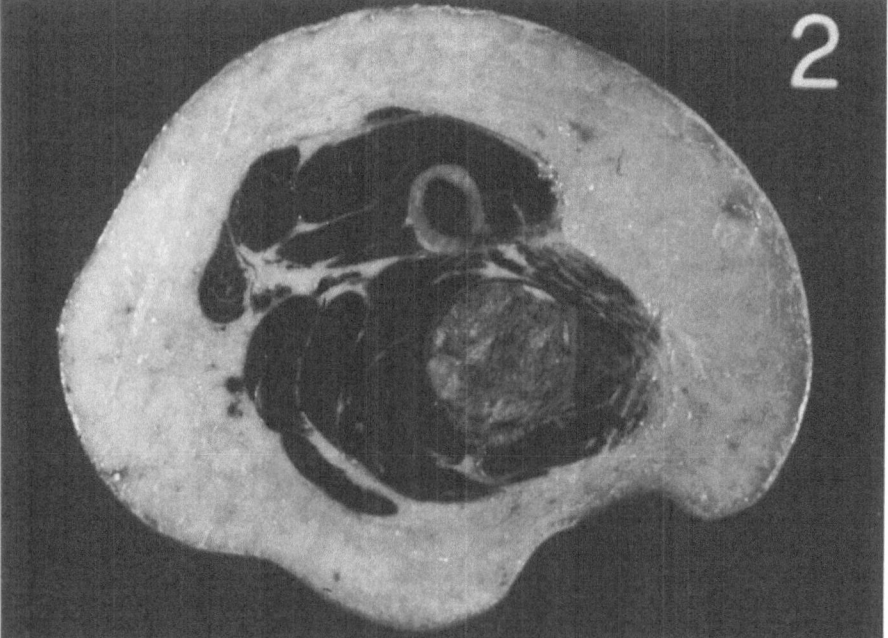

Fig. 1.4. Soft tissue sarcoma of the thigh: specimen. The tumor has a well-developed pseudocapsule but involves numerous muscles in the posterior compartment. The fascia separating the posterior and anterior compartments is a barrier to growth of this tumor from the posterior compartment into the anterior compartment.

barrier to tumor growth; the major fascial boundaries between compartments, however, are not easily penetrated (Fig. 1.4).

The less aggressive benign tumors grow slowly and have such limited invasive properties that, if they penetrate the cortex, a mature periosteal reaction produces a new "expanded" cortex. These lesions do not penetrate cartilage and will not cross major fascial boundaries.

The more aggressive benign tumors and less aggressive malignant tumors will be slowed by the cortex, usually contained by the periosteum, and will not invade cartilage or cross major fascial barriers. Their growth will be more longitudinal than circumferential because there are fewer longitudinal restraints. Their pseudo-capsule, infiltrated by tumor cells, is well developed and easily defined by radiographic and gross histologic methods.

The more aggressive malignant tumors, i.e. those with a high risk of metastasis, rapidly invade the surrounding tissue, penetrating cortical bone and periosteum and crossing fascial boundaries; the cartilage remains a significant barrier though. Vascular channels provide the pathway for local spread across major barriers, as do surgical incisions that violate barriers. The pseudocapsule in these tumors is ill defined, and the surrounding tissue outside the histologically identifiable pseudo-capsule is invaded by tumor cells.

Surgical Staging System

The growth characteristics of musculoskeletal tumors were used in developing a surgical staging system (Enneking et al. 1980). This system is constantly being evaluated and refined, but has proved useful in planning surgical treatment. It is based on the histologic grade of the tumor, its extent, and the presence of metastases (Table 1.1.)

Table 1.1. Basis for staging of musculoskeletal tumors

Grade	G_0 = Benign
	G_1 = Low-grade, malignant
	G_2 = High-grade, malignant
Anatomic extent	T_0 = Intracapsular
	T_1 = Extracapsular, intracompartmental
	T_2 = Extracapsular, extracompartmental
Metastasis	M_0 = Not present
	M_1 = Present

Histologic Grade

Benign tumors are classified as grade 0. Malignant tumors are either grade 1 (G_1, low-grade), if their histologic appearance suggests little risk of metastasis, or grade 2 (G_2, high-grade), if there is a significant risk of metastasis.

Anatomic Extent and Surgical Compartments

To define the anatomic extent of musculoskeletal tumors the concept of compartments has been introduced. The extremities can be considered as divided into
numerous compartments separated by natural barriers to tumor extension. These
barriers are penetrated only by the more aggressive tumors, unless their violation
by surgical incision provides a pathway for tumor growth. The periosteum is a
natural barrier, as is the articular cartilage; therefore, each bone is a single compartment. Muscle groups are separated by thick fascial barriers with little or no vascular
connection that also restrict the growth of tumors. Such muscle groups in the
extremities can therefore also be considered as compartments. Anatomic sites
without natural boundaries are known as primary extracompartmental anatomic
sites (Table 1.2).

The tumor's anatomic extent is classified as either intracompartmental or extracompartmental (Table 1.2). Some tumors originate in primary extracompartmental
sites, but extracompartmental tumors are usually those that have crossed a major
barrier, while intracompartmental tumors are confined to their compartment of
origin. The extracompartmental tumors have the worse prognosis and require more
extensive surgery.

Table 1.2. Anatomic sites of musculoskeletal tumors (T)

Intracapsular (T_0)	Extracapsular, intracompartmental (T_1)	Extracapsular, extracompartmental (T_2)
Intracapsular, intraosseous	Extracapsular, intracortical	Extracortical extension
Intracapsular, intra-articular	Extracapsular, intra-articular	Extra-articular extension
Intracapsular, skin-subcutaneous	Extracapsular, skin-subcutaneous	Deep extension
Intracapsular, parosseous	Extracapsular, parosseous	Extension into bone or soft tissue
Intracapsular, whether intracompartmental or extracompartmental	Extracapsular, intracompartmental soft tissue	Extracompartmental soft tissue Extracapsular, by extension or origin
	Intracompartmental by origin: Ray hand Ray foot Posterior calf ⎫ Separated by Anterolateral leg ⎬ major fasciae Anterior thigh ⎫ Medial thigh ⎬ Separated by Posterior thigh ⎭ major fasciae Buttocks Volar forearm ⎫ Separated by Dorsal forearm ⎬ major fasciae Anterior arm ⎫ Separated by Posterior arm ⎭ major fasciae Deltoid Periscapular	Extracompartmental by origin: Midhand, dorsal or palmar Mid or hind foot Popliteal fossae Periarticular knee Femoral triangle Obturator foramen, pelvis Sciatic notch, intrapelvic Antecubital fossae Periarticular elbow Axilla Periclavicular Paraspinal, head neck

Surgical Stage

Benign tumors are classified as grade 0, and their stage is either 1, 2, or 3, depending on their apparent aggressiveness as revealed by radiologic examinations, or the extent of invasion as seen by histologic examination (Table 1.3). Stage 1 benign neoplasms are those that are least active, do not invade their capsule and usually heal spontaneously. Stage 2 benign neoplasms are active lesions which have minimal invasion of their pseudocapsule and do not escape their structure of origin. These tumors may penetrate the cortex but are contained by the periosteum. Stage 3 is the most aggressive benign category. These lesions invade their pseudocapsule and may extend beyond their structure of origin. Stage 3 bone tumors usually escape the periosteum to involve the surrounding normal tissue, and stage 3 soft tissue tumors are often extensively infiltrative.

The stage of malignant tumors is determined by both the histologic grade and anatomic extent (Table 1.3). Malignant neoplasms without a metastasis are staged as: stage IA (low-grade intracompartmental), stage IB (low-grade extracompartmental), stage IIA (high-grade intracompartmental), or stage IIB (high-grade extracompartmental). Tumors with metastasis are stage III and may be further classified as A or B if desired, although the patient's prognosis and treatment are usually not affected by the local anatomic extent if there is metastatic disease at the first presentation.

The stage of a tumor cannot be finally determined until it has been biopsied, but usually the histologic diagnosis is suspected with a high degree of certainty and the tumor can be presumptively staged on the basis of clinical and radiologic findings prior to the biopsy.

Table 1.3. Surgical stages of musculoskeletal tumors

Benign

Stage 1	$G_0 T_0 M_0$
Stage 2	$G_0 T_0 M_0$
Stage 3	$G_0 T_{1-2} M_0$

Malignant

Stage I

A: Low-grade, intracompartmental	$G_1 T_1 M_0$
B: Low-grade, extracompartmental	$G_1 T_2 M_0$

Stage II

A: High-grade, intracompartmental	$G_2 T_1 M_0$
B: High-grade, extracompartmental	$G_2 T_2 M_0$

Stage III

A: Either grade, intracompartmental, distant metastasis	$G_{1-2} T_1 M_1$
B: Either grade, extracompartmental, distant metastasis	$G_{1-2} T_2 M_1$

References

Enneking WF, Spanier SS, Goodman MA (1980) A system for the surgical staging of musculoskeletal sarcoma. Clin Orthop 153: 106–120

Enzinger FM, Weiss SW (1983) Soft tissue tumors. CV Mosby, St. Louis, p 9

Robbins SL, Cotran RS (1979a) Pathologic basis of disease, 2nd edn. WB Saunders, Philadelphia, p 141

Robbins SL, Cotran RS (1979b) Pathologic basis of disease, 2nd edn. WB Saunders, Philadelphia, p 159

Chapter 2
Surgical Principles

Surgery in a patient with a musculoskeletal neoplasm is indicated either for diagnostic biopsy or for therapeutic resection. Occasionally the two procedures are combined and an excisional biopsy is done. Such a biopsy is appropriate when the preoperative evaluation suggests that the tumor is an aggressive benign (stage 2 or 3) or low-grade intracompartmental (IA) lesion. The margin of the excision should be wide, and the patient's function not adversely affected by the resection. This usually is appropriate for small, well-circumscribed soft tissue lesions situated in the subcutaneous tissue or in a single muscle. A subcutaneous lesion should be removed with a 1–2 cm margin of normal tissue and not just "shelled out." An intramuscular lesion should be excised by removing the entire muscle. Excisional biopsy is also suitable for small cortical or periosteal bone lesions which can be excised without a segmental resection of the bone being required. It is impossible to do a frozen section on many bone lesions, and it is often better widely to excise the lesion on the basis of the clinical and radiologic diagnosis than to perform an incisional biopsy and contaminate tissue unnecessarily. The indications for an excisional biopsy are limited, though, and the procedure must be planned as carefully as any other surgical resection.

Biopsy

An incisional biopsy should be the last step in the evaluation of the patient, undertaken after careful planning. It can usually be done in conjunction with the definitive surgical procedure. When the preoperative evaluation points to a specific diagnosis, both a biopsy with a frozen section diagnosis to confirm the clinical impression and the definitive surgical resection can be done under the same anesthesia. The biopsy must obtain representative diagnostic tissue from the tumor: if done without careful planning biopsies often provide tissue inadequate for histologic diagnosis, either because there is not sufficient of it or it is unrepresentative. The other problem caused by a poorly done biopsy is that tissue is contaminated unnecessarily, and a patient who would be a candidate for limb salvage is converted to an amputee (Mankin et al. 1982). Using the diagnostic studies to plan the biopsy reduces the risk of these complications.

Musculoskeletal neoplasms are often heterogeneous tumors and the correct diagnosis can only be made when the pathologist sees all of the tissue types. Malignant musculoskeletal tumors usually have areas of necrosis, and a diagnosis will not be possible if only necrotic tissue is acquired at the biopsy. Reviewing the diagnostic studies with the radiologist and pathologist while planning the biopsy will increase the chances of obtaining adequate diagnostic tissue, which in turn will significantly improve the pathologist's interest and accuracy. A frozen section should always be done, even if the definitive surgery is not to be done under the same anesthesia, since it is needed to prove that the tissue is representative. It is very embarrassing to discover two days postoperatively that the tissue is non-diagnostic. Some of the tissue should be preserved for examination with the electron microscope, as many musculoskeletal neoplasms require electron microscopic evaluation for a final classification.

Tissues exposed during the biopsy or contaminated by hematoma or drainage tubes used at the time of the biopsy must be considered as potential sites of tumor cells. If the tumor requires surgical excision, the biopsy tract, drainage tube tract, and all tissues contaminated by hematoma must be excised *en bloc*. The surgeon must therefore plan the excision of the tumor so that the minimum amount of tissue is exposed and all tissues contaminated will be resectable. If an immediate resection is not done, the surgeon must obtain strict hemostasis and place the drainage tubes carefully.

Fine needle aspiration and needle biopsies cause less contamination than open biopsies but still contaminate tissue through which they pass. The improper place-ment of a needle can contaminate vital structures, and needle biopsies must be planned just as carefully as open biopsies. Needle biopsies provide limited tissue for histologic examination but are useful when the diagnosis is expected to be easily made on a small sample and when surgical resection of a tumor is not necessary (i.e. Ewing's sarcoma, myeloma, metastatic carcinoma). The interpretation of needle biopsy and fine needle aspiration specimens requires additional expertise on the part of the pathologist, and the pathologist or cytologist should be consulted prior to the biopsy to ensure that the planned procedure is appropriate.

The skin incision for the biopsy should be longitudinal and placed so as not to compromise any possible definitive resection. Major neurovascular bundles should not be exposed during the biopsy. The dissection should be done through the overlying muscle and not between muscle planes, and while it has to be accepted that the biopsy will contaminate adjacent structures, contamination must be minimized and confined to tissue which may be subsequently resected.

The surgeon assuming responsibility for the patient's surgical management is best suited to plan the biopsy. Referring physicians are more likely to make a mis-take and should resist the temptation to do a biopsy before referring the patient.

Definitive Surgery

The majority of musculoskeletal neoplasms are treated by surgical resection. The surgeon must strike the correct balance between removing sufficient tissue to ensure local control and saving sufficient tissue so that the patient will have a functional extremity. As a rule he should err on the side of removing too much tissue, because usually the treatment of a local recurrence leads to a greater functional loss than does a small extra margin of safety.

The preoperative examinations are critical in planning the surgical procedures. The surgeon must know the exact anatomic extent of the lesion in order to determine accurately what must be removed and what can be saved. If a biopsy has been done prior to the radiologic evaluation, the tissue contaminated by the biopsy must be identified so that the surgical incision will include it with the resected specimen. Specific questions which must be answered include: Does the soft tissue tumor invade the adjacent bone? Is the tumor immediately adjacent to the bone, or is there a plane of normal tissue between the bone and soft tissue tumor? Is the soft tissue tumor confined to a single muscle or other compartment, or has it crossed a compartmental barrier? What is the relationship between the tumor and the neurovascular bundle? What is the medullary extent of the bone tumor? Has the bone tumor escaped the cortex or periosteum? Is the adjacent joint involved? And, finally, is there evidence of metastasis? When these questions have been answered the surgical resection can be planned.

To plan the surgical procedure the surgeon must first determine the stage of the tumor. Although the final staging depends upon the histologic grade of the tumor and therefore cannot be definitively assigned until the biopsy is interpreted, in the majority of cases the histologic diagnosis and grade are reasonably certain and a tentative stage based on radiologic and clinical findings can be assigned prior to the biopsy. Once the tumor has been staged the required surgical margin is selected; the more aggressive the tumor the greater the margin required for local control. Surgical margins can be intralesional, marginal, wide or radical (Figs. 2.1 and 2.2) (Enneking et al. 1980).

An *intralesional margin* results from a surgical procedure in which the tumor is removed from within the capsule or pseudocapsule. All incisional biopsies are intralesional procedures as are all curettages. This type of procedure exposes the operative field to gross tumor, and is adequate treatment only for stage 1 benign tumors.

A *marginal margin* is obtained when excision is through the reactive tissue which surrounds the tumor and makes up the pseudocapsule. Tumor cells within the pseudocapsule (satellites) will be left in the patient. This surgical margin is appropriate for stage 1 tumors and is usually sufficient for stage 2 tumors.

A *wide margin* is obtained when the resection includes the tumor surrounded by a cuff of normal non-reactive tissue. This is sometimes called an *en bloc* resection. We would not stipulate a particular measurement of normal tissue which must be included around the tumor, but do believe that more tissue should be included in the longitudinal plane than in the circumferential plane: the natural barriers to tumor growth will restrict it circumferentially, while it is unrestricted longitudinally either within the medullary canal or within a muscle. When practicable, muscles are removed from origin to insertion and as much bone as possible is resected. A wide resection is appropriate surgical treatment for stage 2, 3, IA, IB and some IIA tumors.

A *radical margin* is achieved when the entire compartment involved is removed. This is the safest surgical margin for all neoplasms and is appropriate treatment for stage IIA and IIB tumors. Most radical margins are achieved with an amputation, but some anatomic sites lend themselves to non-amputative radical resection, most notably the anterior thigh (Fig. 2.2).

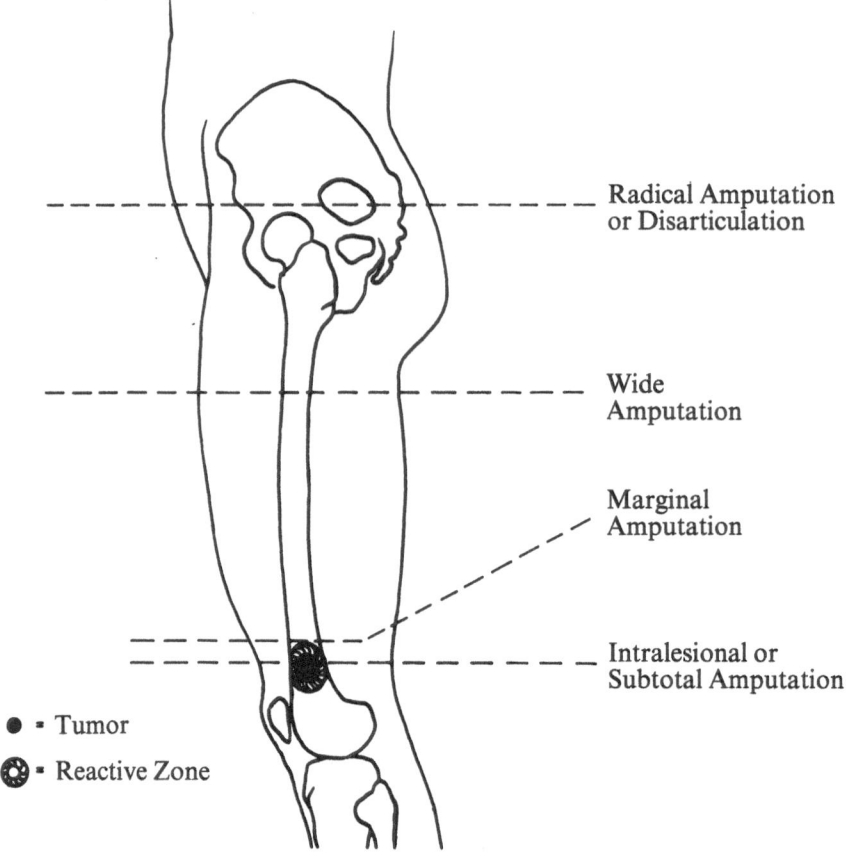

Fig. 2.1. Examples of surgical margins at amputation. An amputation is not necessarily adequate surgery and may result in any surgical margin. (From Enneking et al. 1980, with permission.)

Once the surgical margin required has been established, the surgeon can decide exactly what tissue needs to be resected. The method of reconstruction can then be selected on the basis of what tissue has been left. Limb salvage is possible if the neurovascular supply to the distal tissue is preserved.

The final decision regarding the exact surgical procedure to be used must take the patient into consideration, as each patient has different expectations and limitations. Limb salvage is more demanding both physiologically and financially than amputation, and often the amputee is more active than a patient who has had a limb salvage procedure. The appropriate use of limb salvage surgery is still being defined. Often the utility and advantage of the limb after the resection of a major portion of the bone and/or muscle are only psychological and cosmetic.

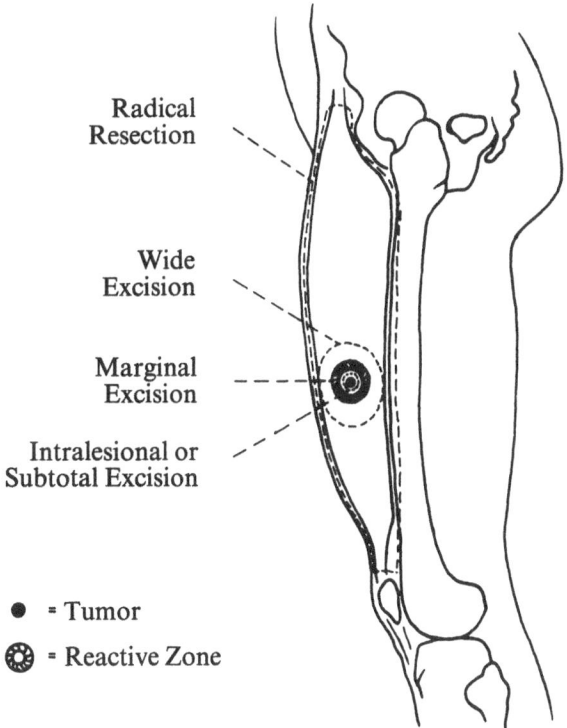

Radical
Resection

Wide
Excision

Marginal
Excision

Intralesional or
Subtotal Excision

● = Tumor

◉ = Reactive Zone

Fig. 2.2. Examples of surgical margins at local procedure (resection). (From Enneking et al. 1980, with permission.)

References

Enneking WF, Spanier SS, Goodman MA (1980) A system for the surgical staging of musculoskeletal
    sarcoma. Clin Orthop 153: 106–120
Mankin HJ, Lange TA, Spanier SS (1982) The hazards of biopsy in patients with malignant primary
    bone and soft-tissue tumors. J Bone Joint Surg [Am] 64: 1121–1127

Chapter 3
Radiologic Evaluation: General Remarks

As described in the previous chapter, modern surgery has changed the demands on the radiologic examination to a considerable degree during the last 10 or 15 years. Commensurately, there have been remarkable developments in the radiologic modalities and procedures, as will be discussed in the next chapter. This has meant that the protocols, technical procedures, and the information gained by radiology today are in many respects different from those of only a decade ago. Three aspects of musculoskeletal tumors should be evaluated radiologically: the local behavior of the tumor, the diagnosis, and the local extent.

Local Behavior of the Tumor

For planning of treatment, and especially of surgery, assessment of the local behavior of the tumor is mandatory. This assessment entails evaluation of the local aggressiveness, which should be distinguished from the histopathologic concepts of benign and malignant. The local aggressiveness can be accurately assessed radiologically for most bone tumors and some soft tissue tumors, and the tumors classified on this basis as either latent, active, or aggressive (Enneking 1983). This classification can, in the majority of cases, be made from the radiologic and clinical appearance of the tumor before the histology is known, as will be discussed and exemplified in Chapter 5.

In *latent lesions* the cells are cohesive and do not infiltrate the capsule or surrounding normal tissue. Such lesions grow very slowly, often resolve spontaneously, and usually do not require treatment. Latent lesions in the soft tissue have a true capsule which the tumor cells do not invade, while those in the bone are surrounded by a well-defined reactive rim of bone. They are usually recognized by the clinical setting and appearance on a plain film radiograph. Latent lesions are benign stage 1.

Active lesions may distend or deform their pseudocapsule but do not extend beyond the reactive rim which surrounds the lesion. They may require surgical treatment since they do not resolve spontaneously but continue to grow. They have an intermediate growth rate and the reactive tissue is capable of containing the lesion. Active bone lesions can erode the cortex but do not penetrate the periosteum, which is usually able to maintain a rim of reactive bone surrounding the tumor. They do not infiltrate the marrow but resorb it, producing a narrow transition zone between the tumor and the normal marrow. Active lesions may be benign stage 2 or occasionally low-grade malignant (stage I).

Aggressive lesions invade and penetrate the capsule and extend into the surrounding reactive and/or normal tissue. Aggressive bone lesions will penetrate the cortex and periosteum with invasion of the surrounding muscles. Cortical destruction may be complete or permeative. They quickly extend into the medullary canal, infiltrating well beyond the border suggested by the plain film radiograph, and often stimulate a wide reactive zone. Aggressive lesions are usually high-grade malignant (stage II), but both low-grade malignant (stage I) and benign processes (stage 3) may present with a highly aggressive pattern. Aneurysmal bone cyst, giant cell tumor, osteomyelitis and eosinophilic granuloma are examples of benign processes which often have an aggressive growth pattern.

In the following chapters we will use the concepts latent, active and aggressive to describe the local behavior of tumors. But in the radiologic literature much effort has been made to differentiate malignant and benign tumours on the basis of the local behavior of the lesions. Therefore, when referring to literature we will also use the terms benign and malignant.

Radiologic Diagnosis

The diagnosis is important, both for planning of treatment, including chemotherapy and/or radiotherapy, and for prognosis. But the definitive diagnosis is a histopathologic concept, and in the preoperative work-up the diagnosis, often based on radiologic findings, can only be made with some degree of uncertainty. The certainty of the diagnosis may be anything from almost certain, with very few differential possibilities (which is most often the case, especially for bone tumors), to a very uncertain suggestion with several possible differential diagnoses. But for the planning of surgery the histopathologic diagnosis is less important than the local behavior and extent of the tumor as evaluated radiologically.

Local Extent

If the tumor is regarded as active or aggressive, and thus surgery is indicated, a detailed depiction of the local extent of the lesion must be obtained. Local recurrence of aggressive benign lesions may threaten the limb, and local recurrence of malignant tumors means a considerably worsened prognosis. To avoid recurrence the tumor must be removed with a safe margin. Therefore, the radiologic work-up must define to which compartment(s) the lesion is confined and whether there is direct contact or overgrowth to adjacent structures such as bone, vessels, nerves or joints.

The Radiologic Assessment as the Basis for Clinical Management

In Chapters 5, 6 and 7 we will discuss the radiologic approach from three main points of view—local behavior, radiologic diagnosis, and local extent—in the order they should be analyzed in the routine clinical setting. Given these three parameters, the surgical staging as described in Chapter 2 can be performed, and the biopsy or definitive surgery planned. But it should be borne in mind that there is a continuum from very latent to highly aggressive lesions, and in individual cases the local behavior, as assessed radiologically, may be uncertain. Moreover, the diagnosis may be uncertain or wrong in a small percentage of cases. Therefore, the clinical decision as to the management of the patient must always be based on a synthesis of all known data: clinical, laboratory, radiologic, and histopathologic. Even though the radiologist should always aim at an assessment that is as precise as possible, the estimation of the final "truth" might be altered by other findings. As a cornerstone in the preoperative work up of musculoskeletal tumors, radiology is indispensable, but a building cannot rest only upon one cornerstone.

Reference

Enneking WK (1983) Musculoskeletal tumor surgery. Churchill Livingstone, Edinburgh, pp 69–168

Chapter 4
Diagnostic Imaging Modalities: Technical Comments

During the last two decades important technologic developments have taken place within diagnostic imaging. For examination of musculoskeletal tumors, the image quality of plain film radiography has increased, mainly due to better film–screen combinations and magnification techniques. Pharmacoangiography, improvements in catheter material, new contrast media and digital techniques have increased the information available with angiography. Following the introduction of ^{99m}Tc-labelled compounds bone scintigraphy has become one of the main methods for evaluation of both benign and malignant musculoskeletal lesions, and the development of modern gamma cameras in combination with advanced computer technology has considerably increased the information that can be gained from this modality. Ultrasonography has had an impact on the evaluation of soft tissue and juxta-articular lesions. Finally, and again mainly because of modern computer technology, computed tomography and magnetic resonance imaging have revolutionized the diagnostic work-up of musculoskeletal tumors.

In this chapter we will discuss technical considerations in the use of the different modalities. The technology behind the modalities will be mentioned briefly, and the possibilities and limitations inherent in the methods will be further discussed in the following chapters, as will their relative diagnostic value.

Conventional Radiography and Tomography

In spite of modern technology, *plain film radiography* remains the basis for radiologic evaluation of musculoskeletal tumors in general, and bone tumors in particular. For accurate assessment of bone destruction and bone reaction, high-resolution systems are necessary, and today most commercial film–screen combinations provide options for fine-detail examinations.

As in all radiographic examinations, anteroposterior and lateral projections are mandatory, and for evaluation of cortical destruction of the long bones several further projections may be taken to cover the circumference tangentially (Wilner 1982).

The information may be increased by magnification techniques—either optical or direct radiographic. For *optical magnification* industrial-type films or film–screen combinations as used in mammography may be used. These provide such high spatial resolution that the finest details are best assessed using an optical device such as a magnification glass or projection on a screen. This technique may be applied to the peripheral parts of the extremities. However, there is seldom need for the method since the spatial resolution achieved with conventional film–screen combinations is sufficient. For the more proximal parts of the body optical magnification becomes less feasible, as the radiation dose increases considerably and the image quality declines because of decreased geometric sharpness and increased scattered radiation. For this part of the body *radiographic magnification* is more suitable. To achieve such magnification a microfocus X-ray tube with a focal spot of about 0.1 mm is used. A geometrical magnification of 2–4 times is achieved by increasing the distance between the patient and the film and decreasing the distance between the tube and the patient. The technique has been used for both primary and metastatic lesions, especially in the axial skeleton, ribs and pelvis (Genant 1981a).

Conventional tomography has in most cases been replaced by computed tomography and magnetic resonance imaging, but may still be used for evaluation of cortical breakthrough of a joint surface or for detection of a nidus in an osteoid osteoma or matrix calcification in cartilaginous tumors (Hudson and Hawkins 1981). Preliminary plain films must always be available so that the most informative plane can be chosen. Hypocycloidal tube motion provides the thinnest sections with most detail in the image. Zonography with thick sections was used in the past for delineation of soft tissue tumors, but nowadays has been replaced by computed tomography or magnetic resonance imaging.

Arthrography

Arthrography may supply additional information to the other modalities on juxta-articular or intra-articular lesions (DeSmet and Neff 1982; Hudson et al. 1984; DeSmet et al. 1985). When a possibly malignant tumor is examined, the needle injection site should be carefully chosen so that the needle tract can be removed *en bloc* with the tumor if intra-articular tumor is found (DeSmet and Neff 1982). It is also advisable to inject a dye into the puncture canal when the needle is withdrawn, to make the canal easily identifiable during surgery and in the specimen. Joint fluid should be aspirated and examined for malignant cells.

Single contrast examination is preferred in most lesions, but double contrast (contrast medium and air) may be advantageous for examination of bone lesions that penetrate the joint or periosteal lesions that are intra-articular (DeSmet et al. 1985). If double contrast examination is performed, only a moderate amount of air should be used in order to minimize the risk of synovial rupture. We routinely use meglumine diatrizoate 60% as contrast medium, but if the patient is in distress metrizamide (Amipaque, Nyegaard AS, Oslo, Norway) reduces discomfort during and after the examination. The new non-ionic contrast media (Iohexol, Iopamidol) should be used as soon as they are released for general use by the national drug authorities. The addition of epinephrine into the joint is advisable in order to lengthen the intra-articular persistence of contrast medium.

If plain film arthrography fails to provide definite answers, and especially if there is a possibility of cortical and cartilaginous breakthrough, tomography should be used in addition. DeSmet et al. (1985) found conventional tomography most suitable for the wrist and the ankle, and also for the elbow and knee when cartilaginous breakthrough was suspected. They preferred computed tomography for the shoulder and hip and for examination of the joint recesses around the elbow and knee.

Angiography

Irvin F. Hawkins, Jr.

Angiography has long been invaluable in the assessment of musculoskeletal tumors (Hudson et al. 1975, 1981, 1983; Ekelund et al. 1977; Hudson and Hawkins 1981). However, with the advent of high-resolution computed tomographic scanning and more recently magnetic resonance imaging, the indications for angiography have become more specific. Today, its most important applications in the diagnostic work-up arise when there is difficulty in visualizing the proximity of the tumor to the neurovascular bundle prior to non-ablative surgery or when there is a question of a vascular lesion, such as an arteriovenous malformation, an angiolipoma or a cavernous venous hemangioma (Fig. 4.1). While of decreased significance in the diagnostic work-up, angiography has, however, assumed an increasingly important role in therapeutic interventional applications such as embolization and chemotherapeutic infusion.

Choice of Catheters

Without a detailed knowledge of angiographic techniques much of the valuable information to be gained from this invasive modality may be sacrificed. For the last 15 years we have used very small catheters for all angiographic studies at our center, including those on bone and soft tissue (Hawkins 1972; Hawkins et al. 1979). In over 1500 cases of bone and soft tissue tumors only one significant complication has occurred. Small catheters have also become increasingly important lately in the light of new therapeutic applications (chemotherapy and embolization) (Jaffe et al. 1985) and economic pressure for more out-patient procedures. We use the small 4.1 French polyethylene Cook catheters, which are very soft, follow the guide wire very easily, and permit directional changes with the use of a deflector. This latter capability is especially useful when catheterizing a contralateral common iliac artery and its distal branches.

Examination of the Upper Extremity

In the past we insisted on antegrade injections in bone and soft tissue angiography to permit good opacification, but for the last 10 years we have found them unnecessary, at least in the upper extremity. A 3 French multiholed catheter with a 0.018 in. end hole and a 40 cm maximum length will deliver 5 ml/s with very little retrograde

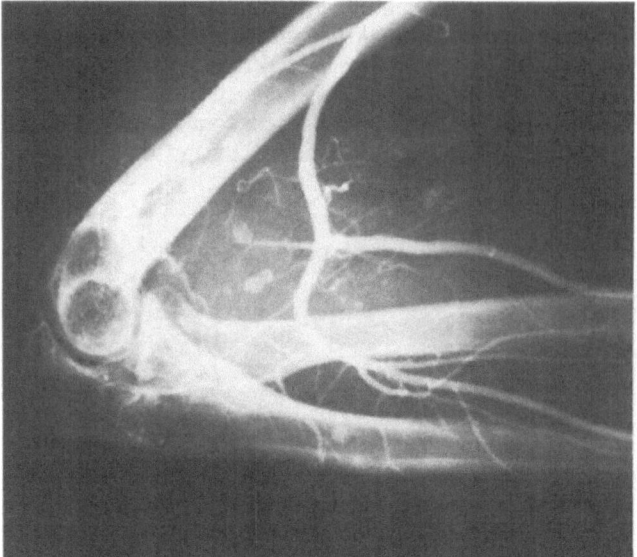

a

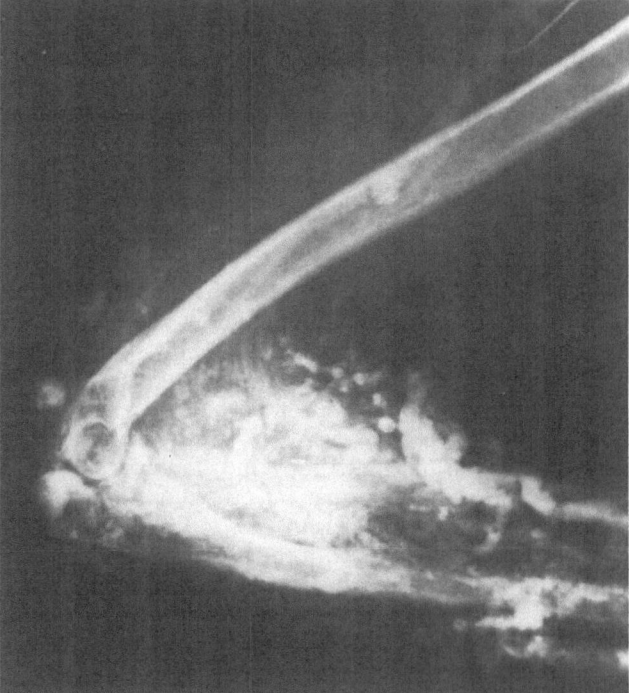

b

Fig. 4.1a,b. Standard film–screen arteriogram. Female, 40 years, cavernous venous hemangioma. Diffuse soft tissue mass of the elbow, forearm and upper arm. Antegrade injection of meglumine diatrizoate 60% after 1 ml of intra-arterial Priscoline with a 4F catheter at 4 ml/s × 6 s for a total of 24 ml: **a** arterial phase, **b** venous phase. Note multiple calcifications on the arterial phase. The arterial phase is normal, while the venous phase shows extensive cavernous venous hemangioma. Using no vasodilator and standard amount of contrast medium the venous changes were not seen.

reflux. We normally inject in the shoulder 5 ml/s for a total of 30 ml (Table 4.1).
If more than 5 ml/s is required, a high-flow 3 French catheter will deliver approximately 7 ml/s of meglumine diatrizoate 60%. For the upper extremity we normally
use meglumine diatrizoate 60% without intra-arterial xylocaine, since xylocaine
may cause cerebral depression. If the vasodilator tolazoline (Priscoline, Ciba-Geigy
Corp., USA) is used (Hawkins and Hudson 1974; Ekelund et al. 1977) one should
inject it very slowly to avoid reflux into the cerebral circulation. Usually 12.5–25 mg
of Priscoline is injected intra-arterially and very slowly approximately 1 min before
the injection of contrast medium. We prefer the brachial artery approach since
there is no danger of brachial plexus injury which can occur with axillary puncture.
We prefer the brachial approach to the femoral also, since it eliminates traversing
the brachiocephalic vessels (diminishing the possibility of stroke) as well as prevent-
ing inadvertent catheter recoil into the cerebral circulation. Films are always
obtained in several projections to delineate clearly the proximity of the tumor to
the major vessels.

Table 4.1. Angiographic technique

Injection site	Standard film–screen combination + meglumine diatrizoate 60%	Digital subtration angiography + arterial meglumine diatrizoate 60%	CO_2 angiography
Upper extremity	3F catheter (brachial) 5 ml/s × 6 s total 30 ml	3F (brachial) 3–4 ml/s × 6 s total 18–24 ml	CO_2 contraindicated
Abdomen	4F (femoral) 15 ml/s × 3 s total 45 ml	3F (femoral) 4 ml/s × 4 s total 16 ml	3F (femoral) 10 ml/s × 8 s total 80 ml
Pelvis (selective)	4F (fem. contralat.) 6–8 ml/s × 6 s total 36–48 ml	3F (fem. ipsilat.) 3 ml/s × 5 s total 15 ml	3F (fem. ipsilat.) 4F (fem. contralat.) 10 ml/s × 5 s total 50 ml
Lower extremity	4F (fem. contralat.) iliac: 9 ml/s × 6 s total 54 ml femoral: 6–8 ml/s × 6 s total 36–48 ml popliteal: 5–6 ml/s × 6 s 30–36 ml	3F (fem. ipsilat.) 2–3 ml/s × 6 s total 12–18 ml	3F (fem. ipsilat.) 4F (fem. contralat.) 10 ml/s × 5 s total 50 ml

Examination of the Retroperitoneum and Pelvis

For a retroperitoneal tumor, an aortogram is obtained using a high-flow 4 French
catheter which will deliver approximately 15 ml/s. An injection of 15 ml/s for 3 s
is usually made in the anteroposterior and possibly oblique positions. If lumbar
arteries are supplying the tumor, selective injections are made with a 4 French
shepherd's Cook catheter.

For pelvic tumors, initially a distal aortic injection is made, usually with a high-flow catheter injecting 15 ml/s for a total of 3 s. Films are obtained in the antero-posterior projection. Depending upon the arterial supply, either a common iliac or an external or internal iliac injection is then made. Usually the pelvic arteries are approached contralaterally, since it is very easy to advance a catheter into the contralateral internal iliac artery with the use of a tip deflector. In an average patient usually 6 ml of meglumine diatrizoate is injected for a total of 6 s, again using a vasodilator (Priscoline 25 mg) (Table 4.1). Films are obtained in multiple projections in an attempt to delineate the extent of the tumor.

Examination of the Lower Extremity

For most tumors of the lower extremity we prefer the contralateral approach using a 4 French catheter and tip deflector to position the catheter in the contralateral common iliac artery. A long 0.028 in. J-guidewire can very easily be advanced as far as the trifurcation, and the small, soft catheter will readily follow (Fig. 4.2). The injection rates decrease as the catheter is more distally positioned in the pelvis

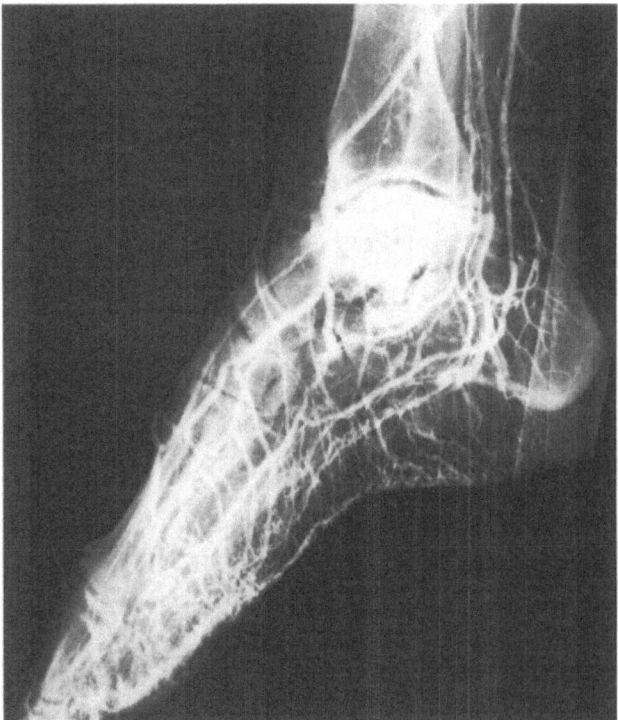

Fig. 4.2. Standard film–screen arteriogram. Male, 40 years, giant cell tumor of the talus. Late arterial phase of antegrade popliteal injection, 6 ml/s of meglumine diatrizoate 60% × 6 s for a total of 36 ml after the infusion of 1 ml Priscoline. Note the good filling of the small vessels of the entire foot. There is a homogeneous blush in the talus.

and leg. In the common iliac artery, 9 ml/s for a total of 6 s is injected. In the common femoral artery, normally 6–8 ml/s is injected. In the popliteal area, usually 5–6 ml/s is injected, again depending upon the size of the tumor and vessel (Table 4.1). Usually 25 mg of Priscoline is used, with a repeat dose of half the initial dose if multiple injections are made. A blood pressure cuff inflated above systolic pressure and placed distal to the tumor may also improve the study, since less contrast is "lost" to the distal distribution and distal pain is eliminated.

Analgesia

Using standard film–screen angiography, large volumes of contrast medium are necessary to obtain a good capillary and venous phase, which accurately delineates most lesions. When ionic contrast media are used these large volumes make the study extremely painful. In adults and children older than about 12 years, we have found the most effective premedication to be Valium (10–15 mg orally) in combination with Dilaudid (1.5–2.0 mg intramuscularly). Such premedication, when combined with a mixture of 2 mg of 2% xylocaine per millilitre of contrast medium, provides studies in which the patient is not caused to move due to pain and the discomfort is tolerable. For children under 12, general anesthesia is advisable.

It is to be hoped that in the near future this analgesic regimen will be obviated by the use of arterial digital subtraction angiography (DSA), or non-ionic compounds or carbon dioxide as the contrast medium. Arterial DSA permits reduced injection rates of ionic contrast agents, producing only a warm sensation and occasional discomfort in the patient. The use of non-ionic contrast media with DSA should completely eliminate the discomfort (Mills et al. 1982; Widrich et al. 1982; Nyman et al. 1983). In our experience with carbon dioxide as a contrast medium, less than 10% of patients experienced any discomfort in a series of over 300 cases (Hawkins 1985).

Digital Subtraction Angiography (DSA)

Intravenous DSA has not been used extensively for the study of bone and soft tissue tumors. However, in young patients who have good cardiac output and a higher probability of arterial spasm and possible occlusion, intravenous injections have been very helpful in several cases (Fig. 4.3). Normally we inject 1.5 ml/kg with a venous catheter positioned in either the right atrium or the caval vein (superior caval vein after antecubital approach, and inferior caval vein after femoral approach).

For arterial DSA a 3 French catheter can be placed retrograde in the femoral, brachial or axillary arteries, and usually 3–4 ml/s of meglumine diatrizoate for a total of 6 s gives excellent opacification (Table 4.1). Although the detail is not as good as with a film–screen combination, the tumor blush in the case of vascular tumors is usually better, and the venous phase is also excellent.

DSA enables the use of even smaller catheters and reduces the amount of contrast medium. This increases safety while minimizing discomfort. With further technical improvement of the digital system, resolution should approach that of standard film–screen techniques.

Carbon Dioxide Angiography

We have used carbon dioxide as a contrast medium in over 150 bone and soft tissue tumors (Hawkins 1985). In most cases the results have been comparable to those of standard arteriography. In vascular tumors the tumor blush is usually better seen with iodinated contrast; however, the extent of the tumor can usually be well visualized with carbon dioxide (for the doses used see Table 4.1). We found that a high percentage of malignant tumors demonstrated shunting with carbon dioxide which was not seen with standard iodinated contrast material (Fig. 4.4) (Hawkins 1985).

Carbon dioxide has the advantage of permitting the use of very small catheters (3 French). It also eliminates the risk of allergic reactions, presents no apparent danger of renal or hepatic toxicity, and causes either no or only very minimal discomfort. Furthermore, as a contrast agent it is very inexpensive. It should be stressed that we use carbon dioxide only for examination of the pelvis and legs; it is contraindicated for examination of the arms because of the risk of cranial embolization.

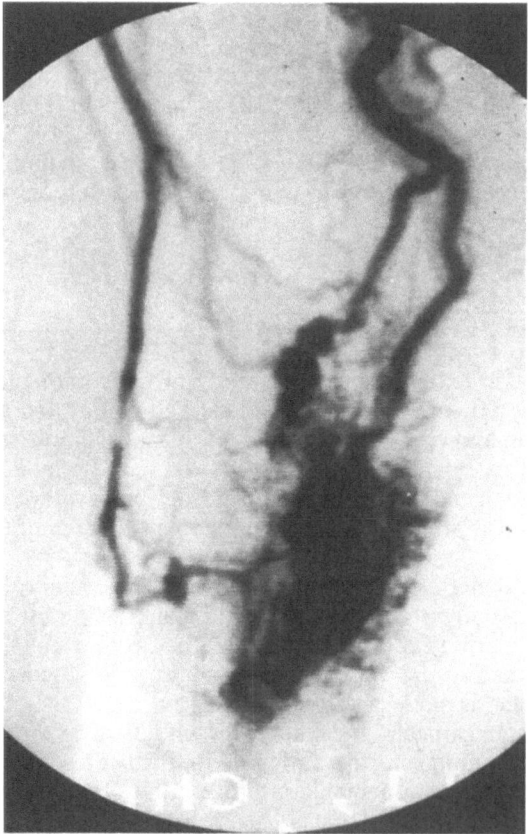

Fig. 4.3. Digital subtraction angiography (DSA). Female, 25 years, arteriovenous malformation. Venous DSA (25 ml/s × 2 s of meglumine diatrizoate 60% into the right atrium) demonstrates a vascular mass in the plantar surface of the foot with large feeding arteries and draining veins.

Xeroradiography

Xeroradiography using selenium as photoconductor is a radiographic application of the xerographic process as first described by Carlson in 1937 (Genant 1981b). It has two characteristic features: edge enhancement and a broad latitude. The edge enhancement means that borders between areas of different densities are sharply demarcated even if the density difference is small. The broad latitude means that structures with high density, such as bone, and low density, such as fat, are all well depicted on one and the same image. The method has been used for evaluation of soft tissue tumors (Bernardino et al. 1981), but for evaluation of the tumor matrix within bone it is inferior to plain film examination. Today, the method is only seldom used for evaluation of musculoskeletal tumors.

Ultrasonography

Diagnostic ultrasound using sonic waves with a frequency between 2 and 10 MHz has achieved an important position in diagnostic imaging during the last 10 years. However, for examination of patients with musculoskeletal tumors its role is limited (Kobayshi et al. 1975; deSantos and Goldstein 1977). Although solid and cystic soft tissue masses can be differentiated, the local behavior of a tumor cannot be evaluated and there is little information as to the diagnosis (Scheible 1981). Ultrasonography has been successfully used for follow-up during radio- or chemotherapy, and it may be helpful in localizing soft tissue masses for percutaneous biopsy (Holm et al. 1975).

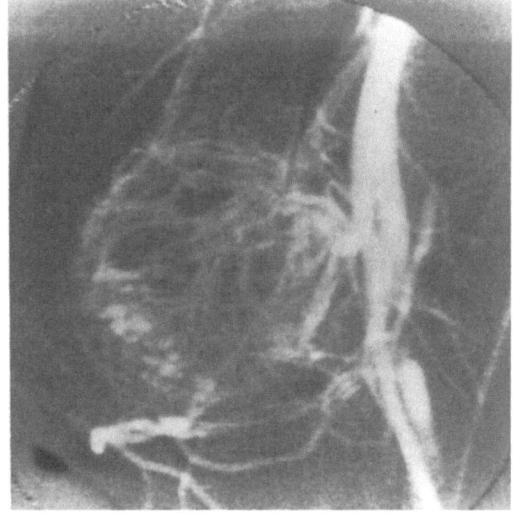

Fig. 4.4. Carbon dioxide angiography. Male, 16 years, osteosarcoma. Early arterial phase shows the popliteal and genicular arteries feeding a large vascular tumor with a soft tissue mass extending to within 1 cm of the vascular bundle. The popliteal vein opacified almost immediately as a result of arteriovenous shunting.

Scintigraphy

Bone scintigraphy has been available for more than 25 years, but because of the high radiation dose, early methods using ^{85}Sr (Bauer and Ray 1958; Bauer and Wendeberg 1959) were feasible mainly for the diagnosis of metastases in patients with known malignant disease. With the advent of ^{99m}Tc-labelled bone-seeking substances in the early 1970s and, later, ^{67}Ga, and with the development of modern gamma cameras, the radiation load on the patient has decreased considerably, while the information on musculoskeletal disease has increased dramatically. Today, bone scintigraphy is one of the mainstays in orthopedic radiology for examination of both benign and malignant conditions.

The most commonly used agent for examination of patients with musculoskeletal tumors is ^{99m}Tc-labelled methylenediphosphonate (^{99m}Tc-MDP), but several other inorganic pyrophosphates and polyphosphates or organic phosphonates may also be used. With modern camera systems the dose of ^{99m}Tc-MDP injected should be 15–20 mCi for adults, equivalent to about 8 mCi/m^2 body surface in children (Gilday et al. 1977). Also ^{67}Ga has proved to be of value, especially for examination of soft tissue tumors. The dose of ^{67}Ga used for adults is 3–5 mCi.

If whole body images are routinely obtained, spot films of the diseased area are mandatory. With modern sensitive detection systems the entire examination may be performed with spot films of different anatomic areas, the sum of the spot areas covering the whole body.

To allow the size of musculoskeletal tumors to be assessed, for instance the intraosseous extent of tumor, radioactive markers should be placed immediately adjacent to the extremity or part of the body examined (Fig. 4.5). This is important if the scintigraphic results are to be used for the planning of surgical resection. In examination of soft tissue tumors it is important that several different projections are taken of the lesion—not only anteroposterior and lateral but also oblique projections—to evaluate the relation between the tumor and adjacent bone (see Chapter 7).

Computed Tomography (CT)

Following the development of the first clinically useful CT scanner in 1970 (Hounsfield 1973) and the recognition of its enormous potential, CT technology rapidly evolved.

CT has three great advantages over conventional radiography: (1) high contrast resolution, (2) cross-sectional imaging with the possibility of reconstruction in other planes, and (3) the capability of measuring attenuation values. Today, CT is an indispensable tool in any well-equipped department of radiology. The technique has revolutionized diagnostic imaging and has had a great impact on the diagnostic approach to musculoskeletal tumors during the last 10 years. Potentials and limitations of CT in this patient group are fairly well established today, and even though the techniques used during the examination may vary, certain basic rules can be given.

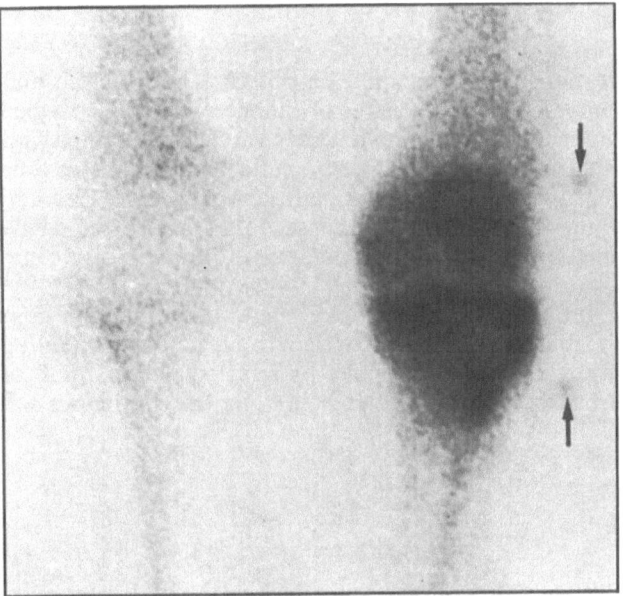

Fig. 4.5. Radiographic markers for scintigraphy. Female, 24 years, giant cell tumor of the tibia. The markers (^{57}Co; *arrows*) are placed immediately adjacent to the limb at a known distance apart (in this case 10 cm) to allow measurement of the size and extent of tumor.

Patient Position and Choice of Sections

The patient should be placed on the CT table as comfortably as his or her condition allows, but still so that the optimum possible alignment is obtained between the plane of the CT sections and the anatomic planes. If repeat examinations are performed, for instance during radio- or chemotherapy, it is important that the patient be positioned as nearly as possible in an identical position each time and that the same sections are obtained.

All modern scanners have equipment for digital radiography and a preliminary digital radiograph covering the area to be examined as well as neighboring anatomic landmarks must be obtained. Even though the spatial resolution does not equal that of a conventional radiograph, the anatomic landmarks and the lesion itself will be identified, and the region to be scanned can be defined (Fig. 4.6a,b). The digital radiograph also acts as a perfect localization system in the analysis of findings, since any changes seen in the transverse sections can be localized and related to the anatomic landmarks on the digital radiograph (Pettersson and Harwood-Nash 1982) (Fig. 4.6b,c).

Transaxial sections with 10 mm slice thickness are the rule, but thinner sections may be advantageous in small lesions and in or near the joints. In selected cases, especially in children, direct frontal or sagittal sections may be performed (Kaiser et al. 1981). Reconstruction in the frontal or sagittal plane is possible with all modern machines. To obtain a clinically acceptable reconstructed image, continuous, thin (1.5–5 mm) transaxial sections must be obtained, but even so the resolution is only moderate (Fig. 4.6f).

Contrast Medium Infusion

If there are no contraindications, images should be obtained both before and during/after contrast medium injection. The degree of enhancement may be a clue to diagnosis and may also inform the surgeon of a widely vascularized tumor with potentially large blood loss during surgery. Thus, we routinely take three or four sections at different levels through the lesion before infusion of contrast medium. Then, during contrast medium infusion, continuous sections through the whole lesion are obtained, including apparently normal tissue both proximal and distal to the tumor (Fig. 4.6d,e).

For contrast medium we use 60% meglumine diatrizoate; the total adult dose is 200 ml and in children it is adjusted according to weight to a maximum of 3 ml/kg body weight. The contrast medium is administered by infusion, the first half of the total dose being given before and the second half while the continuous CT

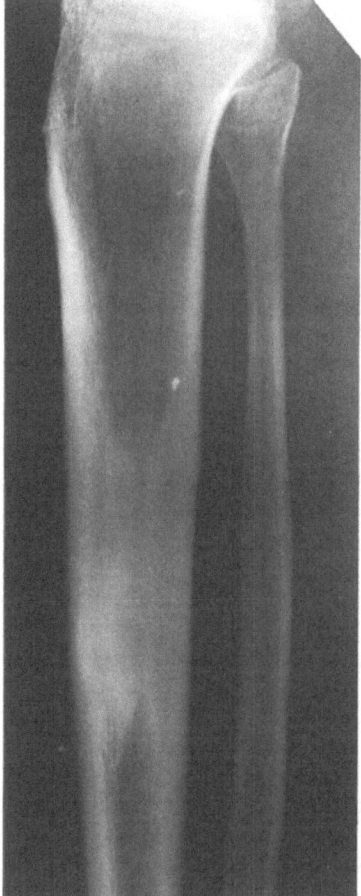

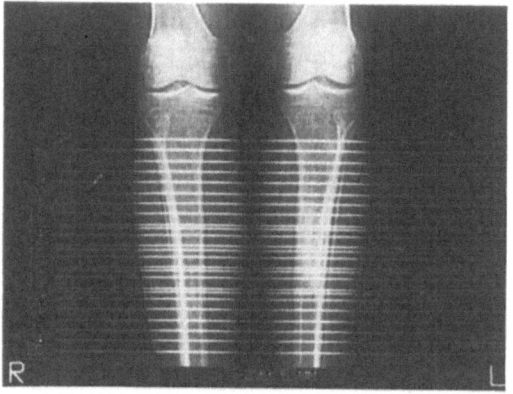

a

b

Fig. 4.6a–f. CT technique. Male, 36 years. a The plain film reveals a dense new bone formation in the shaft of the tibia. b In the digital radiograph the lesion is well visualized. The horizontal cursor lines denote the sections. c Section number 16 in the middle of the lesion shows the dense new bone formation. d and e Sections numbers 9 and 24 are the first proximal and distal slices, respectively, where the bone looks normal, and where the attenuation value in the narrow canal is the same as that in the contralateral side. The numbers to which the arrows are pointing denote the mean attenuation values in the region of interest outlined by the cursor. f Reconstruction in the sagittal plane displays the extent exactly, but with poor spatial resolution.

sections are obtained. We have found infusion to be superior to bolus injection in most cases, since it keeps the concentration of contrast medium high both in the lesion and in the adjacent main vessels. This enables accurate analysis of the relation between the neurovascular bundles and the tumor. If there is need for a detailed definition of the vessels or vascularization of some area, bolus injections are added.

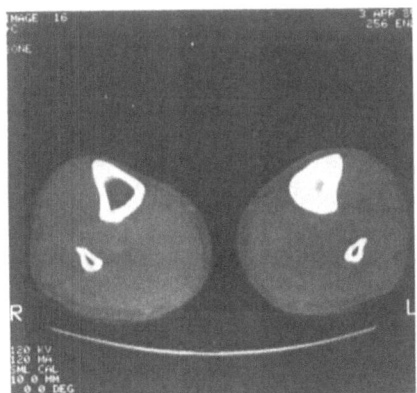

c

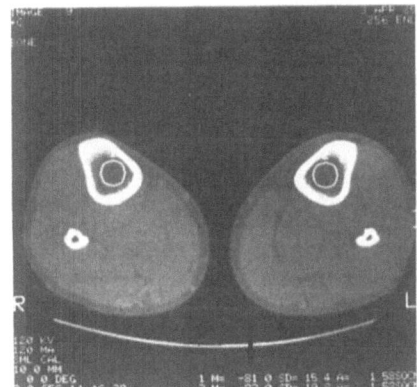

d

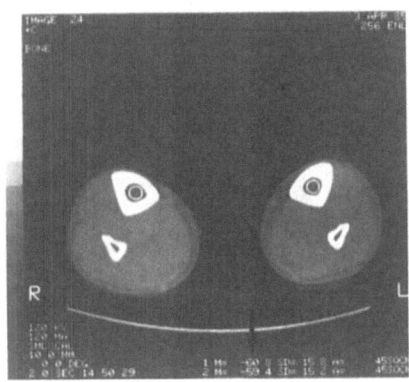

e

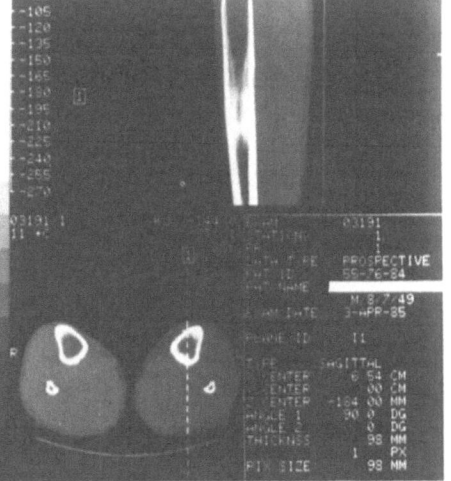

f

Technique for Image Evaluation

Following the study the image should be scrutinized and films should be obtained
with at least two window settings: one with a high window level and width ("bone
window") and one with a low level and width ("soft tissue window") (Fig. 4.7).
Using only one intermediate setting is not acceptable; two settings permit an accurate estimation of both the bone and soft tissue components.

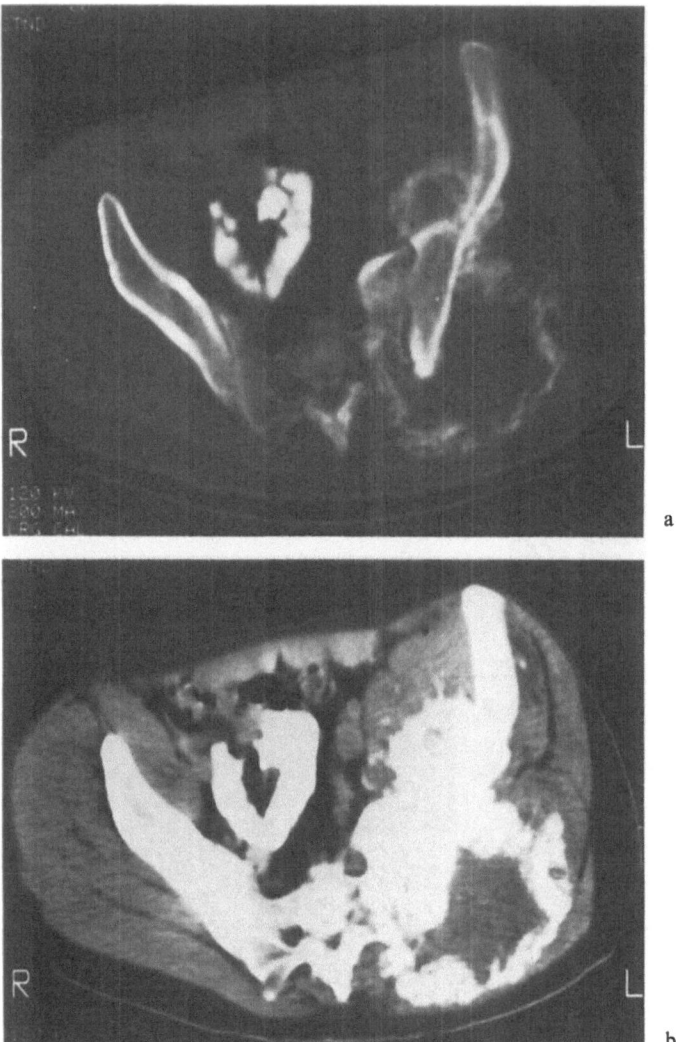

a

b

Fig. 4.7a,b. CT images with "bone window" setting (a) and "soft tissue window" setting (b). Male,
17 years, osteogenic sarcoma after chemotherapy. The "bone window", with a high window level and
width, allows analysis of the skeletal changes, while the "soft tissue window" of the same image, with
a low window level and width, reveals the composition and extent of the soft tissue component.

The attenuation values in the tumor should be measured in the sections taken before contrast medium infusion, to be compared with the values in the same sections during infusion. The "pre-contrast" values may give a clue to the composition of the tumor matrix, as will be discussed in Chapter 6. Also, measuring the attenuation values in the medullary cavity on the diseased and the contralateral side will give an estimation of the intraosseous extent of tumor, as described in Chapter 7. The enhancement during infusion is directly related to the degree of vascularization and, therefore, the degree of enhancement may be used to differentiate highly vascularized tumors from those with low or no vascularization, as discussed in Chapter 6. However, it is obvious that the absolute increase in attenuation varies with the amount of contrast medium given. When an infusion technique is used the increase is therefore dependent upon the time during the period of infusion at which the section was obtained, making absolute values of limited usefulness.

Magnetic Resonance Imaging (MRI)

MRI is based on the phenomenon of nuclear magnetic resonance, which was first described in the 1940s. The basis for the phenomenon is nuclear magnetization caused by the application of strong magnetic fields, and the reorientation and relaxation of this magnetization when intermittent radiofrequency fields of specific frequencies are added. For the imaging of these phenomena advanced computer programs are used, similar to those developed for CT.

Although the use of nuclear magnetic resonance in medical imaging has been available for only a few years, it is obvious that this modality has brought a new dimension to medicine. The main advantages of MRI are that: (1) it has better contrast discrimination than any other modality; (2) imaging in any plane is easily available; (3) it has a potential for tissue characterization based on proton density, T1 and T2 relaxation times, chemical shift and flow (most commercial systems today are based on proton magnetization and proton imaging); and (4) with higher field strength systems, spectroscopic tissue characterization is also possible. For musculoskeletal imaging MRI affords a further advantage: most modern orthopedic procedures and devices have very little or no ferromagnetic capacity (i.e. contain little or no iron) and thus there are no metallic artifacts analogous to those seen with CT (Mechlin et al. (1984).

In orthopedic radiology MRI is already an established modality for examination of spinal disease, aseptic necrosis and musculoskeletal tumors, and it has a proven potential for imaging a wide variety of other conditions (Pettersson et al. 1985a). There are several reports in the literature concerning technique, possibilities and limitations of this method for examination of primary musculoskeletal tumors, and our own experience is based on examinations of about 400 patients with such disease.

In any MRI system good imaging requires optimization of the following parameters: the field strength, the design of the coils (the antennae with which the radiofrequency pulses are transmitted and received), the choice of pulse sequences (the ordering of the radiofrequency pulses which orient the nuclear magnetization), and the imaging plane and slice thickness.

Field Strength

For a short period it was thought that only superconductive systems with moderate or high field strengths of 0.3–1.5 tesla (T) were appropriate for proton imaging, but it has lately become obvious that, given updated software and improved surface coil design (Fitzsimmons et al. 1985; Pettersson et al. 1985a,c), images of excellent quality can be obtained by resistive systems operating at lower field strengths (0.15 T). For ^{31}P-imaging and spectroscopy, high field strengths are necessary, the minimal strength being 1.5–2 T (Nidecker et al. 1985).

Coil Design

Appropriate changes in coil design may dramatically increase the image quality (Fitzsimmons et al. 1985; Pettersson et al. 1985a,c). For imaging of the extremities we have found surface coils of the half-saddle type to be of great advantage, while for imaging of the spine and hips circular surface coils have proved useful. Several of the commercial MRI systems offer options for surface coils, and a set of such coils is very advisable for musculoskeletal imaging.

Pulse Sequences

In medical imaging the most commonly used pulse sequences are inversion recovery (IR), saturation recovery (SR) and spin echo (SE). For musculoskeletal imaging a combination of IR and SE sequences, or only SE sequences, is most commonly used. The IR sequence will give information on the longitudinal (T1) relaxation, while SE sequences may be designed to give information either mainly on T1 relaxation ("T1-weighted images") or on the transverse (T2) relaxation ("T2-weighted images"). SE sequences with short repetition times (TR = 250–500 ms) and short echo times (TE = 30 ms or less) (T1-weighted) depict the anatomy of joint structures, muscles, tendons and fat in great detail. Musculoskeletal tumors in such sequences often have about the same signal intensity as the surrounding muscle (Fig. 4.8a). These sequences, therefore, are apt to delineate intraosseous tumors from the bone marrow and soft tissue tumors from the subcutaneous fat, as the bone marrow and fat have much higher signal intensities. In SE sequences with long TR and TE (TR = 1500–2000 ms, TE = 60–120 ms) (T2-weighted), the signal intensity from most tumors is considerably higher than that from the surrounding tissues, and such sequences are well suited for evaluation of the relation between the tumor and normal surrounding tissue, especially the muscle (Fig. 4.8b–e). We have routinely used SE sequences with TR/TE of 500/30 ms to gain T1 information, and TR/TE of 2000/30, /60, /90, /120 ms for T2 information. The latter sequence has been performed in a multi-echo mode. There are several other possibilities for pulse sequence selection, and the optimal sequence has still to be found.

Imaging Plane and Slice Thickness

For examination of the extremities, the two SE sequences mentioned above are routinely performed in the transaxial plane, with a multislice technique giving 10–15

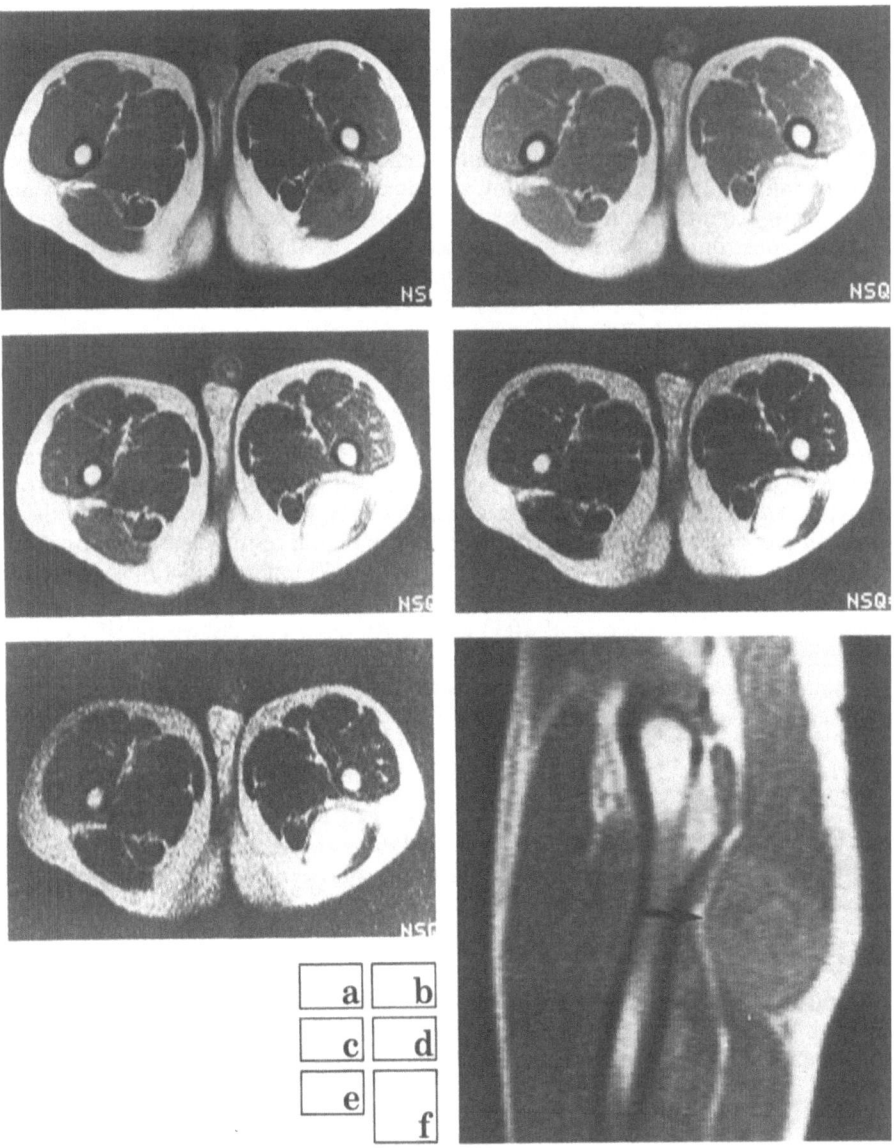

Fig. 4.8a–f. MRI examination technique. Male, 40 years, undifferentiated soft tissue sarcoma of the thigh. Spin echo (SE), multislice multi-echo technique, slice thickness 10 mm. **a** Transaxial section, SE 500/30 ms. **b–e** Transaxial section, 2000/30 (**b**), 2000/60 (**c**), 2000/90 (**d**) and 2000/120 (**e**) ms. **f** Sagittal section, 500/30 ms.

In the T1-weighted transaxial image (**a**) the anatomy of the muscles, bone, fat and vessels is well depicted, while the tumor has about the same signal intensity as the surrounding muscles and is barely visible. In the T2-weighted images (**b–e**) the signal to noise ratio decreases with increasing echo time, but the signal intensity from the tumor is much higher than that from the muscle, giving good delineation of the lesion. The sagittal section (**f**) reveals the longitudinal extension of the tumor as well as the relation between the tumor and the fascia (*arrow*).

contiguous or spaced slices with a slice thickness of 1 cm. This slice thickness could be diminished for evaluation of juxta-articular structures or small lesions. In our routine these two sequences are followed by an additional sequence in the coronal or sagittal plane, or in a plane parallel to the longitudinal axis of the long bone being examined, which provides important information on craniocaudal tumor extent (Fig. 4.8f). For examination of intra-articular lesions or intraosseous lesions with possible breakthrough to the joint, additional sections in the sagittal or coronal planes or in a plane parallel to the long bone may be of advantage. As regards the spine, most information is to be gained from sagittal sections combined with sections perpendicular to the vertebral column or canal.

Calculation of Relaxation Times

Calculations of the T1 and T2 relaxation times using the commercially available imaging systems should be performed with caution, since the values found are dependent upon a great number of variables and are subject to significant errors (Pettersson et al. 1985c, 1986). For such calculations, several methods may be used based on measurements of signal intensity in the region of interest in two or more images (Moon et al. 1983; Pettersson et al. 1985c; Zimmer et al. 1985). We have used three sequences for calculation of T1: the SE 500/30 ms and 2000/30 ms mentioned above and an additional 1000/30 ms. As described elsewhere (Pettersson et al. 1985c) we measure the signal intensity in the same region of interest on these three images obtained from the same section of the body (Fig. 4.9). These data are fitted to an equation of the form

$$I(\text{SE}) = A[1 - \exp(-TR/\text{T1})],$$

where $I(\text{SE})$ is the image intensity, A is the intensity at $TR/\text{T1}$, and TR is the pulse interval. For the T2 calculation we have used data obtained from the same region of interest on the 2000/30, /60, /90, /120 multi-echo acquisition mode, and these data are fitted to an equation of the form

$$I(\text{SE}) = A \times \exp(-TE/\text{T2}),$$

where $I(\text{SE})$ is the image intensity, A is the intensity at $TE=0$, and TE is the echo interval. We have found this method accurate and reproducible, giving an acceptable estimate of T1 (Pettersson et al. 1986; Slone et al. 1986).

NMR Spectroscopy

Most clinical magnetic resonance imagers available today operate at field strengths between 0.15 and 1.5 T and allow only proton imaging. With higher field strengths (1.5–4 T or more), not only protons but also nuclei such as ^{13}C, ^{19}F, ^{23}Na and ^{31}P can be used, which enables a combination of imaging and spectroscopy of the same area to be performed. The first reports of such ^{31}P magnetic resonance spectroscopy of human musculoskeletal tumors in vivo are encouraging (Griffiths 1983; Nidecker et al. 1985), and this method has potential not only for detailed tumor-tissue characterization, but also for evaluation of metabolites developing in the tumor during chemo- and/or radiotherapy.

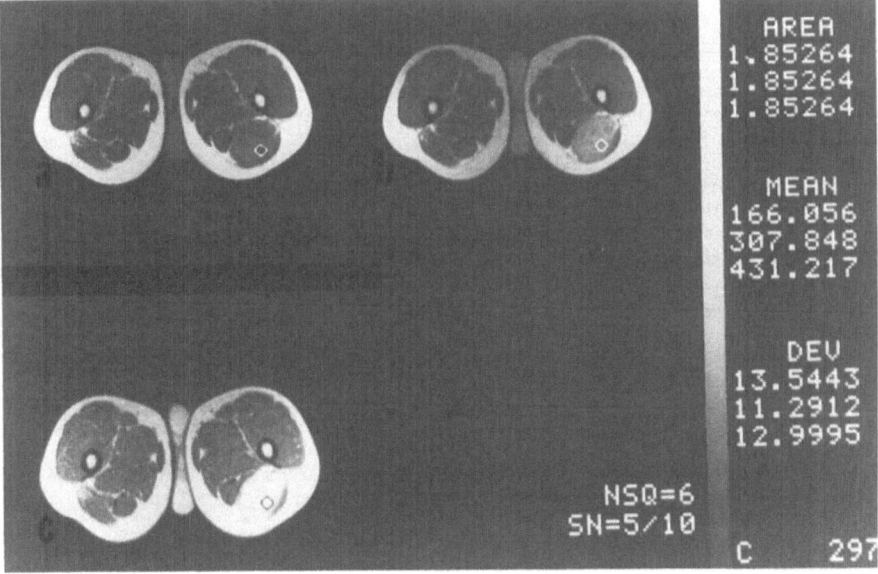

Fig. 4.9a–c. MRI, T1 calculation. Same patient as in Fig. 4.8. The signal intensity is measured in the same region of interest in a set of three images: SE 500/30 ms (**a**), 1000/30 ms (**b**), and 2000/30 ms (**c**). The mean values for the signal intensity are found on the right and they are used for calculation of the T1 value as described in the text. (From Pettersson et al. 1985, with permission.)

References

Bauer GCH, Ray RD (1958) Kinetics of strontium metabolism in man. J Bone Joint Surg [Am] 40: 171–76

Bauer GCH, Wendeberg B (1959) External counting of ^{47}Ca and ^{85}Sr in studies of localized skeletal lesions in man. J Bone Joint Surg [Br] 41: 558–563

Bernardino ME, King BS, Thomas JL, Lindell MM, Zornoza J (1981) The extremity soft-tissue lesions: A comparative study of ultrasound, computed tomography and xeroradiography. Radiology 139: 53–59

deSantos LA, Goldstein HM (1977) Ultrasonography in tumors arising from the spine and bony pelvis. AJR 129: 1061–1064

DeSmet AA, Neff JR (1982) Knee arthrography for the preoperative evaluation of juxtaarticular masses. Radiology 143: 663–666

DeSmet AA, Levine E, Neff JR (1985) Tumor involvement of peripheral joints other than the knee: Arthrographic evaluation. Radiology 156: 577–601

Ekelund L, Laurin S, Lunderquist A (1977) Comparison of a vasconstrictor and a vasodilator in pharmacoangiography of bone and soft-tissue tumors. Radiology 122: 95–99

Fitzsimmons JR, Thomas RG, Mancuso AA (1985) Proton imaging with surface coils on a 0.15T-resistive system. Magn Reson Imaging 2: 180–185

Genant HK (1981a) Magnification radiography. In: Resnick D, Niwayama G (eds) Diagnosis of bone and joint disorders. WB Saunders, Philadelphia, pp 320–345

Genant HK (1981b) Xeroradiography. In: Resnick D, Niwayama G (eds) Diagnosis of bone and joint disorders. WB Saunders, Philadelphia, pp 374–378

Gilday DL, Ash JM, Reilly BJ (1977) Radionuclide skeletal survey for pediatric neoplasms. Radiology 123: 399–406

Griffiths JR, Cady E, Edwards RHT et al. (1983) ^{31}P-NMR studies of a tumour in situ. Lancet I: 1435–1436

Hawkins IF Jr. (1972) "Mini-catheter" technique for femoral run-off and abdominal arteriography. AJR 116: 199–203

Hawkins IF Jr. (1985) CO_2 digital subtraction angiography. Diagn Imaging 7: 82–84

Hawkins IF Jr., Hudson T (1974) Priscoline in bone and soft-tissue angiography. Radiology 110: 541–546

Hawkins IF Jr., Haseman MK, Gelfand PN (1979) Single mini-catheter technique for abdominal aortography and selective injection. Radiology 132: 755–757

Holm HH, Pedersen JF, Kristensen JK, Rasmussen SN, Hancke S, Jensen F (1975) Ultrasonically guided percutaneous puncture. Radiol Clin North Am 13: 493

Hounsfield GN (1973) Computerized transverse axial scanning (tomography). I. Description of a system. Br J Radiol 46: 1016–1020

Hudson TM, Hawkins IF Jr. (1981) Radiological evaluation of chondroblastoma. Radiology 139: 1–10

Hudson TM, Haas G, Enneking WF, Hawkins IF Jr. (1975) Angiography in the management of musculoskeletal tumors. Surg Gynecol Obstet 141: 11–21

Hudson TM, Enneking WF, Hawkins IF Jr. (1981) Value of angiography in planning surgical treatment of bone tumors. Radiology 138: 283–292

Hudson TM, Schiebler M, Springfield DS et al. (1983) Radiologic imaging of osteosarcoma: Role in planning surgical treatment. Skeletal Radiol 10: 137–146

Hudson TM, Schiebler M, Springfield DS, Enneking WF, Hawkins IF Jr., Spanier SS (1984) Radiology of giant cell tumors of bone: Computed tomography, arthro-tomography, and scintigraphy. Skeletal Radiol 11: 85–95

Jaffe N, Robertson R, Ayala A et al. (1985) Comparison of intra-arterial cis-platinum with high dose methotrexate and citrovorum factor rescue in the treatment of primary osteosarcoma. J Clin Oncol 3: 1101

Kaiser MC, Pettersson H, Harwood-Nash DC, Fitz CR, Armstrong E (1981) A direct coronal CT-mode of spine in infants and children. AJNR 2: 465–466

Kobayshi T, Yoh S, Shinohara N, Fukuma H (1975) Echographic diagnosis of soft tissue tumors in extremity and trunk. Jap J Clin Oncol 5: 97

Mechlin M, Thickman D, Kressel HY, Gefter W, Joseph P (1984) Magnetic resonance imaging of postoperative patients with metallic implants. AJR 143: 1281–1284

Mills SR, Wertman DE, Heaston DK et al. (1982) Study of safety and tolerance of iopamidol in peripheral arteriography. Radiology 145: 57–58

Moon KL, Genant HK, Helms CA, Cafetz NI, Crooks LE, Kaufman L (1983) Musculoskeletal applications of nuclear magnetic resonance. Radiology 147: 161–171

Nidecker AC, Muller S, Aue WP et al. (1985) Extremity bone tumors: Evaluation by P-31 MR spectroscopy. Radiology 157: 167–174

Nyman V, Nilsson P, Westergren (1983) Pain and hemodynamic effects in aortofemoral angiography. Clinical comparison of iohexol, ioxaglate and metrizoate. Acta Radiol [Suppl] 366: 171–172

Pettersson H, Harwood-Nash DC (1982) CT and myelography of the spine and cord. Springer-Verlag, Berlin Heidelberg New York, pp 5–21

Pettersson H, Hamlin DJ, Mancuso A, Scott KN (1985a) Magnetic resonance imaging of the musculoskeletal system. Acta Radiol [Diagn] 26: 225–235

Pettersson H, Krop D, Hamlin D, Fitzsimmons J (1985b) Magnetic resonance imaging of the extremities. I. Technique for depiction of normal anatomy. Acta Radiol [Diagn] 26: 299–302

Pettersson H, Krop D, Hamlin D, Fitzsimmons J (1985c) Magnetic resonance imaging of the extremities. II. T1 and T2 relaxation times of muscle and fat. Normal values, reproducibility and dependence on physiologic variations. Acta Radiol [Diagn] 26: 413–415

Pettersson H, Spanier S, Fitzsimmons JR, Slone R, Scott KN (1985d) MR imaging relaxation measurements in musculoskeletal tumors and surrounding tissue. Radiology 157(P): 109

Pettersson H, Hamlin D, Scott KN (1986) MRI of primary musculoskeletal tumors. CRC Crit Rev Clin Radiol Nucl Med (in press)

Scheible W (1981) Diagnostic ultrasound. In: Resnick D, Niwayama G (eds) Diagnosis of bone and joint disorders. WB Saunders, Philadelphia, pp 409–421

Slone RM, Sattin W, Pettersson H, Scott KN (1986) NMR T_1 determination with spin echo sequences. Radiology (submitted)

Widrich WC, Robbins AH, Rommel AJ, Andrews R (1982) Iopamidol: A non-ionic contrast agent for peripheral arteriography. Radiology 145: 53–55

Wilner D (1982) Radiology of bone tumors and allied disorders. WB Saunders, Philadelphia, pp 25–75

Zimmer WD, Berquist TH, McLeod RA et al. (1985) Bone tumors: Magnetic resonance imaging versus computed tomography. Radiology 155: 709–718

Chapter 5

Local Behavior of the Tumor: Growth Pattern and Growth Rate

The local behavior of a tumor is reflected by the rate and pattern of its growth. These can, to a considerable degree, be evaluated radiologically, especially in bone tumors. The true growth rate—i.e. the change in size of a tumor over a period of time—can only be assessed if two or more examinations spaced in time are available (Fig. 5.1). The reason for such repeat examinations may be that the lesion was overlooked on the first occasion, or that it was regarded with a sufficient degree of certainty as benign. In these cases there may be a change not only in size but also in appearance: for instance, in the pattern of calcification in a chondroblastoma or chondrosarcoma (Rosenthal et al. 1984), mineralization of a nidus in an osteoid osteoma, or the formation of "onion peel" periosteal reaction (see below) in a Ewing's sarcoma. Repeat examinations may then give a clue both to the aggressiveness of the tumor and to the diagnosis (Wilner 1982).

In most cases, however, the radiologist has to determine the local behavior from examinations performed on only one occasion. For bone tumors especially, this is possible with a high degree of accuracy (Lodwick et al. 1980a,b), while for soft tissue tumors the possibilities are more limited (Springfield et al. 1984).

Bone Tumors

In bone tumors, changes related to growth pattern and rate of growth can best be regarded from two aspects: bone destruction and bone reaction (Wilner 1982). Most information is gained from plain film radiography, but scintigraphy and, to some degree, CT may also be important for evaluation of the tumor.

Bone Destruction as Seen in the Plain Film Examination

Bone destruction is the most common feature of bone tumors. The plain film appearance of this has been classified by Lodwick (1966a,b) into geographic, motheaten, and permeative. A *geographic* lesion is a large, well-circumscribed "hole" in the bone. The term is used regardless of the shape of the lesion and the type

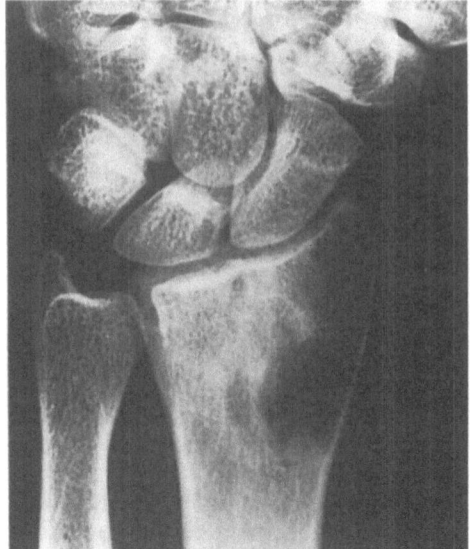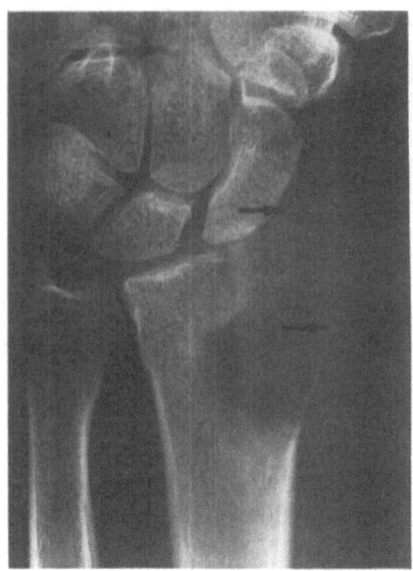

a   b

Fig. 5.1a,b. Growth rate of tumor assessed by repeat examinations spaced in time. Female, 21 years, recurrence of giant cell tumor. At diagnosis of the recurrence (**a**) there is a radiolucent lesion in the distal radius, with preserved cortex. The patient chose to postpone the treatment for social reasons. Two months later (**b**) the aggressive tumor has destroyed part of the cortex (*between arrows*) and the radiolucent area is considerably larger.

of zone between the lesion and surrounding normal tissue. Thus, geographic destruction may be round and "punched-out" with a sharp border as in eosinophilic granuloma (Fig. 5.2), or irregular with a ragged border as in an active giant cell tumor (Fig. 5.3). In *moth-eaten* destruction there are multiple small lytic areas that are often confluent. If the cortex is involved, its outline will be partially destroyed. Metastatic disease of the bone is a typical example of this pattern (Fig. 5.4). In *permeative* destruction the involved area contains numerous very small lytic lesions, so small that even if the cortex is involved, its gross outline is preserved. This pattern is common in round cell tumors such as reticulum cell sarcoma or Ewing's sarcoma (Fig. 5.5). Often, the geographic and other patterns of destruction coexist in the same tumor (Fig. 5.4). It may be difficult or even imposible to distinguish between the moth-eaten and permeative patterns; therefore, Lodwick has modified his classification so that these two patterns are categorized together (Lodwick et al. 1980b).

Classification according to Lodwick

Lodwick (1971) has demonstrated a general correlation between the pattern of destruction and the rate of growth, geographic destruction being consistent with slow growth, permeative with the most rapid growth, and moth-eaten with an intermediate growth rate. But it is also clear that the appearance of the bone reaction

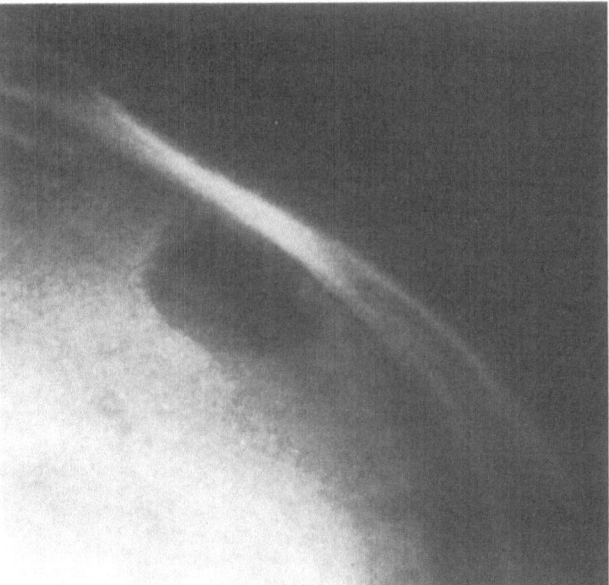

Fig. 5.2. Geographic destruction. Male, 30 years, eosinophilic granuloma. The osteolytic lesion in the skull is rounded with a sharp border.

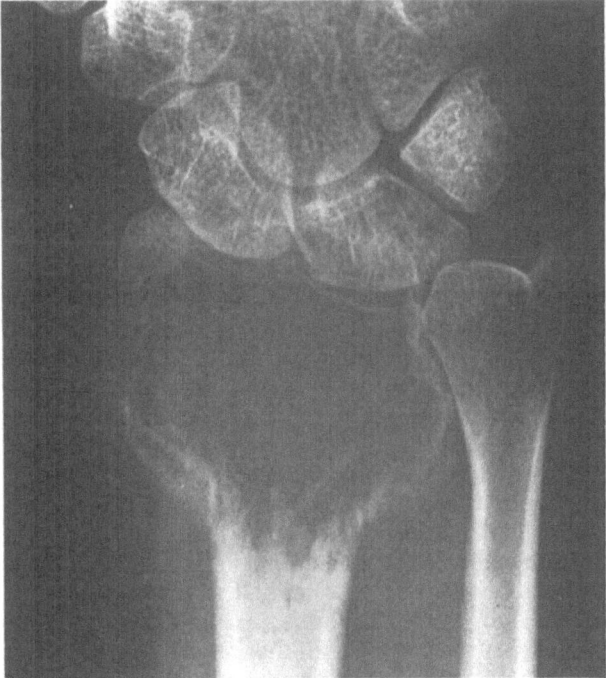

Fig. 5.3. Geographic destruction. Female, 26 years, giant cell tumor. The cortex is expanded and the border between the radiolucent lesion and the normal cancellous bone is irregular and "ragged."

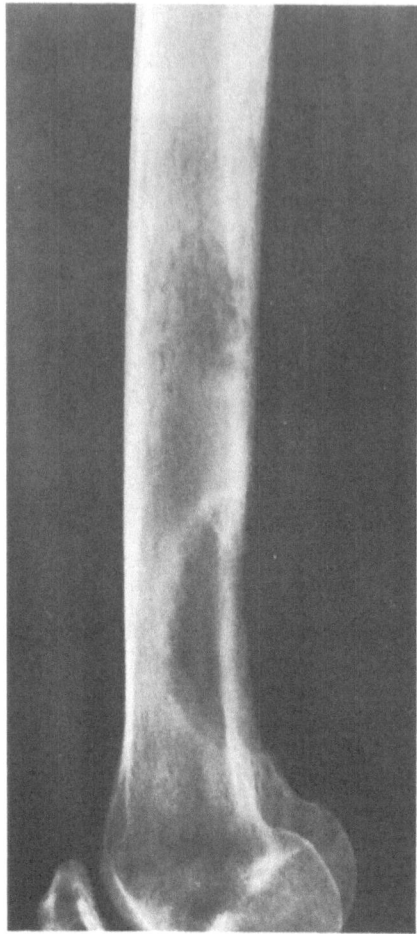

Fig. 5.4. Geographic and moth-eaten destructions. Male, 71 years, metastasis from renal cell carcinoma. The geographic destruction in the distal femoral shaft is well defined. Proximal to this there is a region with multiple small lytic areas, involving the cortex.

in the zone between the lesion and the normal skeletal tissue gives valuable additional information as to growth rate. Lodwick has therefore created a classification based on both the pattern of destruction (including cortical penetration) and the bone reaction, mainly expressed as the presence or absence of a "sclerotic rim" around the lesion and the presence or absence of an "expanded shell" of cortex (these changes will be discussed below) (Table 5.1). The grades in this classification give a good estimate not only of the growth rate, but also of the malignancy of the lesion. In general, the survival rate decreases with an increasing grade (Lodwick et al. 1980a), but grade IB and IC lesions have similar survival rates as have grades II and III lesions. (Note that these grades are different from those in the surgical staging system.) However, for modern surgical planning it is more important to classify a lesion as to its local behavior rather than its degree of malignancy. Therefore, a simplified radiologic classification may be used that categorizes lesions into latent, active, and aggressive stages. Such a classification must be based on both the bone destruction as defined by Lodwick and a detailed analysis of the bone reaction.

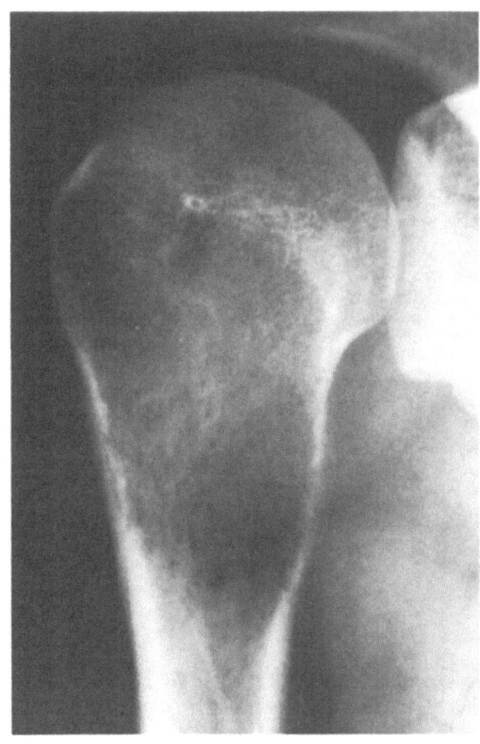

Fig. 5.5. Permeative destruction of the humeral metaphysis and upper diaphysis.

Table 5.1. Radiographic grading of the growth rate of musculoskeletal tumors according to Lodwick (from Lodwick et al. 1980a, with permission)

Radiographic pattern	IA	IB	IC	II	III
Destruction	Mandatory[a] geographic	Mandatory geographic	Mandatory geographic	Moth-eaten or geographic	Mandatory permeated
Edge characteristic	One of 3 patterns: 1. Regular *or* 2. Lobulated *or* 3. Multicentric	One of 4 patterns: 1. Regular *or* 2. Lobulated *or* 3. Multicentric *or* 4. Ragged/poorly defined	One of 5 patterns: 1. Regular *or* 2. Lobulated *or* 3. Multicentric *or* 4. Ragged/poorly defined *or* 5. Moth-eaten 1 cm or less	If geographic, mandatory moth-eaten edge greater than 1 cm	Any edge
Penetration of cortex	None or partial	None or partial	Mandatory total	Total by definition	Total by definition
Sclerotic rim	Mandatory	Optional[b]	Optional	Optional but unlikely	Optional but unlikely
Expanded shell	Optional, only 1 cm or less	If sclerotic rim present, expanded shell must be greater than 1 cm	Optional	Optional but unlikely	Optional but unlikely

[a] Mandatory = essential to the grade.
[b] Optional = may or may not be present.

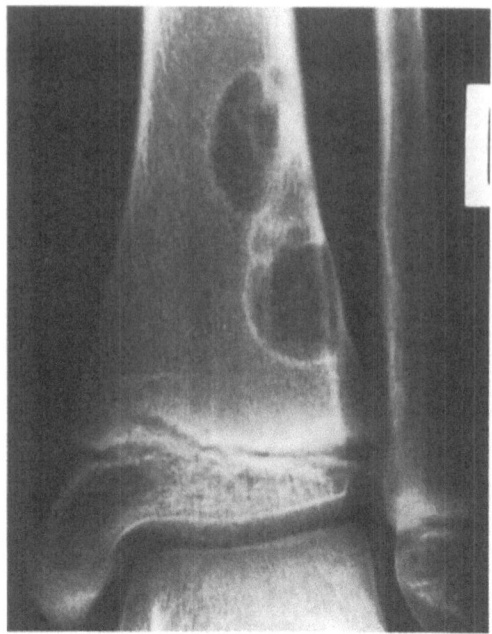

Fig. 5.6. Latent lesion. Male, 14 years, non-ossifying fibroma. The tumor causes geographic destruction, with a very slight expansion of the cortex and a thick cortical "rim" towards the normal cancellous bone. There is no periosteal reaction.

Bone Reaction as Seen in the Plain Film Examination

The expansion of the tumor stimulates a mesenchymal proliferative response in which primitive mesenchymal cells mature to osteoblasts; hence, the reactive zone is composed of maturing bone. This bone reaction represents the local defense mechanism in response to the lesion and is found between the true capsule of the tumor and the normal tissue. The radiologic appearance of this margin varies with the aggressiveness of the tumor (Lodwick 1966a,b; Madewell et al. 1981).

In *latent lesions* (as defined in Chapter 3) the reactive bone slowly forms a continuous, thick capsule of cortical bone around the entire tumor. Trabeculae of bone may extend from this shell through the true fibrous capsule of tumor and into the lesion (Fig. 5.6).

In *active lesions* there may also be a cortical capsule formed around the tumor, but not necessarily. If there is a cortical capsule it will be thin, and due to high osteoclastic activity on its inner side and osteoblastic activity on its outer side, it may expand in all directions, resulting in a "bulging shell" that still contains the tumor inside it. While the tumor is expanding through the cortex, the periosteum is preserved, forming new periosteal bone around the lesion (Fig. 5.7). This is the "expanded cortical shell" of Lodwick's classification.

Aggressive lesions have no cortical rim in the reactive zone, and no mature bone is formed in the reactive zone—the mesenchymal bone-forming cells are too rapidly destroyed by the growing tumor from the inside of the zone. If the normal cortex is involved, it is often eroded (Fig. 5.8).

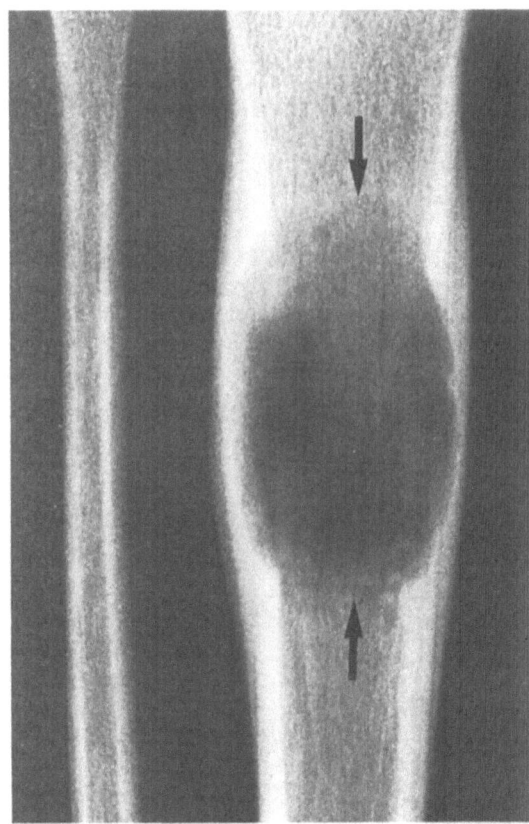

Fig. 5.7. Active lesion. Male, 9 years, eosinophilic granuloma. The tumor has no cortical "rim" towards the normal cancellous bone, but there is a sharp well-defined transition zone (*arrows*). Where the tumor has extended through the cortex, new periosteal bone has formed an "expanded shell."

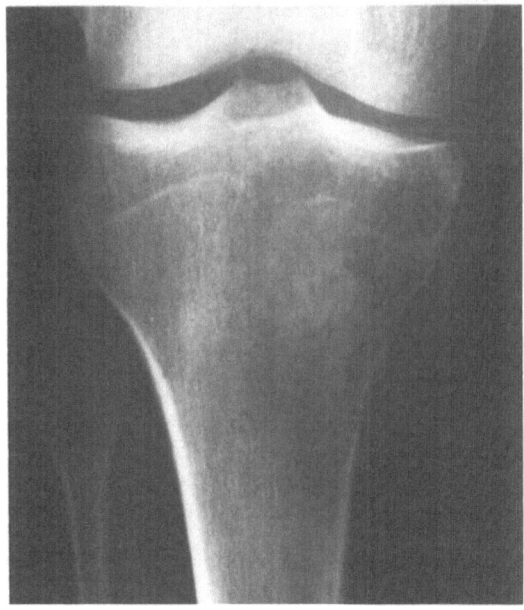

Fig. 5.8. Aggressive lesion. Female, 19 years, osteosarcoma of the proximal tibia. Permeative/moth-eaten destruction of the cancellous bone, with partial destruction of the cortex. The transition zone between the lesion and the normal cancellous bone is wide and ill defined.

Endosteal and Periosteal Reactions

The so-called endosteal and periosteal reactions may also, to some degree, indicate the local behavior of the underlying tumor.

Endosteal Reaction

The endosteal reaction does not differ from the mesenchymal proliferative response to the tumor discussed above, and may appear as a solid thickening of the inner cortex in latent or active lesions (Fig. 5.9), or as mottling throughout the adjacent cancellous bone in aggressive lesions. In aggressive lesions with rapid growth along the medullary canal, there may be remnants of reactive bone on the endosteal aspect of the cortex (so-called buttresses).

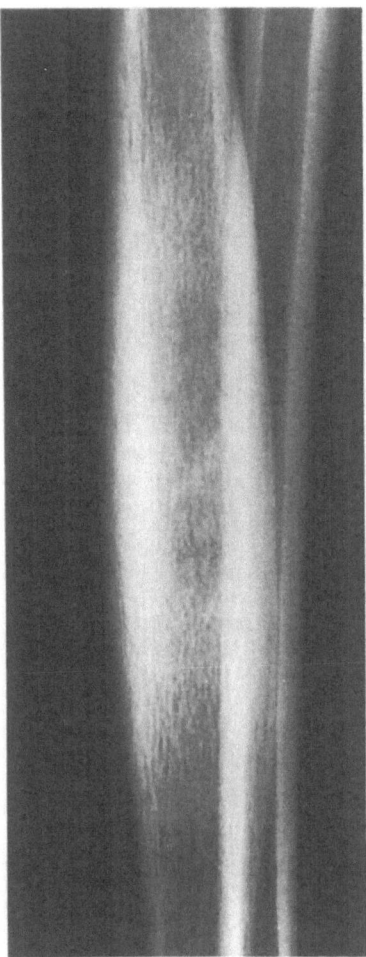

Fig. 5.9. Endosteal reaction. Male, 15 years, osteoblastoma. There is a solid thickening of the endosteal bone, combined with formation of new periosteal bone.

Periosteal Reaction

The fibrous periosteum is richly vascularized, with an inner layer of primitive mesenchymal cells. Numerous perpendicularly oriented collagen fibers connect the cortical bone with the periosteum. The periosteal reaction occurs when the tumor or the reactive rim around it involves the outer surface of the cortical bone (Enneking 1977). A mere "lifting-up" of the periosteum, from subperiosteal bleeding or abscess, is not visible on the plain film radiograph, but the reactive response, with mesenchymal proliferation and bone formation, is clearly seen (Ragsdale et al. 1981; Kricun 1983). The periosteal reaction is usually classified as either solid, lamellated (single or multiple) or perpendicular, and it may also occur as the "periosteal expanded shell" or "Codman's triangle."

The *solid reaction* is composed of one uniform thick layer of bone (more than 1 mm thick) parallel to the cortex and with a thin resolution zone between the cortical bone and the reaction (Fig. 5.10). It is generally seen in latent or active lesions (Edeiken et al. 1966) such as osteoid osteoma and eosinophilic granuloma, but has also been described in association with slow-growing metastases (Norman and Ulin 1969).

The *lamellated reaction* may occur in a thin single layer, as seen in both active benign lesions such as chondroblastoma and aggressive lesions such as Ewing's sarcoma (Garber 1951; Edeiken et al. 1966; Ragsdale et al. 1981). A variation of this is the single, amorphous, thick irregular layer seen, for instance, in aggressive lesions such as round cell tumor and fibrosarcoma (Lodwick 1966b). The reason

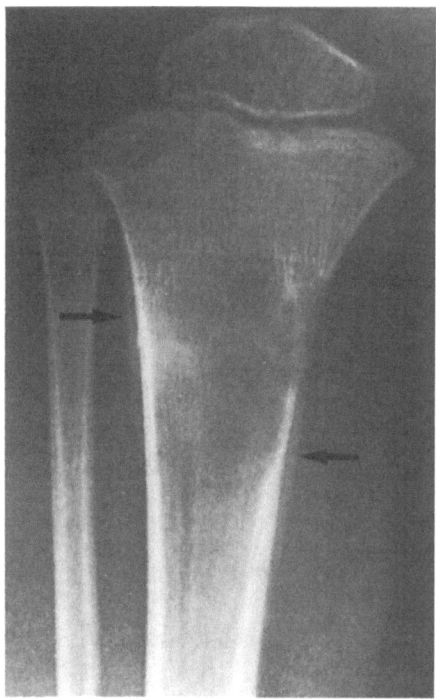

Fig. 5.10. Solid periosteal reaction. Male, 8 years, simple bone cyst with possible fracture. There is a 2 mm thick, solid reaction on both sides (*arrows*), with a thin radiolucent zone between the reaction and the cortical bone.

for multiple concentric layers of ossification ("onion peel") is still not clear, but the most commonly accepted explanation is that it is caused by alternating periods of slow and rapid growth of the tumor, each exacerbation pushing out the periosteum because of attendant edema (Brunschwig and Harmon 1935) (Fig. 5.11).

The *perpendicular (spiculated) periosteal reaction* is caused by bone formation along the fibrous strands and vessels connecting the cortical bone and the uplifted periosteum (Enneking 1977). The radiologic appearance of this reaction may vary considerably and has many descriptive names—for instance "sunburst" or "sunrise" (Kricun 1983) (Fig. 5.12). Even though some of the patterns are more often seen with certain tumors, such as osteosarcoma or Ewing's sarcoma, the variation is so wide that in the individual case the pattern is not diagnostic (Wilner 1982). This reaction is seen with aggressive lesions that have a rapid growth rate and generally with primary malignant tumors or metastases (Nelson 1966).

The *periosteal expanded shell* (Fig. 5.13), described in most textbooks as a periosteal reaction (Edeiken 1981; Wilner 1982), represents merely the expanding cortical capsule around an active lesion, as discussed above.

"*Codman's triangle*" is seen when a rapidly growing tumor has penetrated the cortex and the only remnants of the mesenchymal reaction from the periosteum are small triangles of reactive bone at the proximal and distal extent of the breakthrough (Lodwick 1966b; Ragsdale et al. 1981) (Fig. 5.12). Once "Codman's triangle" was regarded pathognomonic for malignant tumors, but it is now well recognized that it may occur with a variety of non-neoplastic lesions that lift up the periosteum (Kricun 1983).

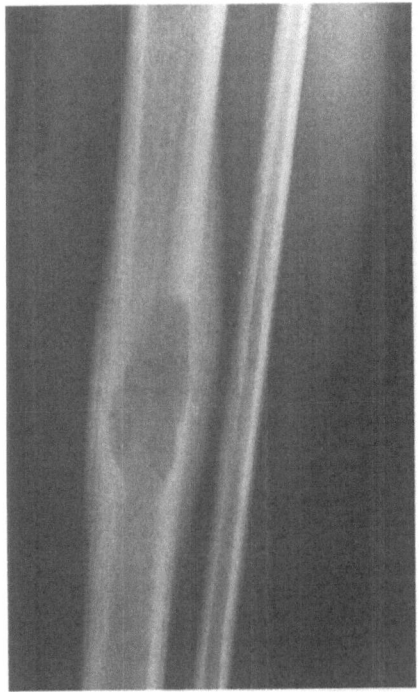

Fig. 5.11. Lamellated periosteal reaction. Male, 10 years, eosinophilic granuloma of the tibia.

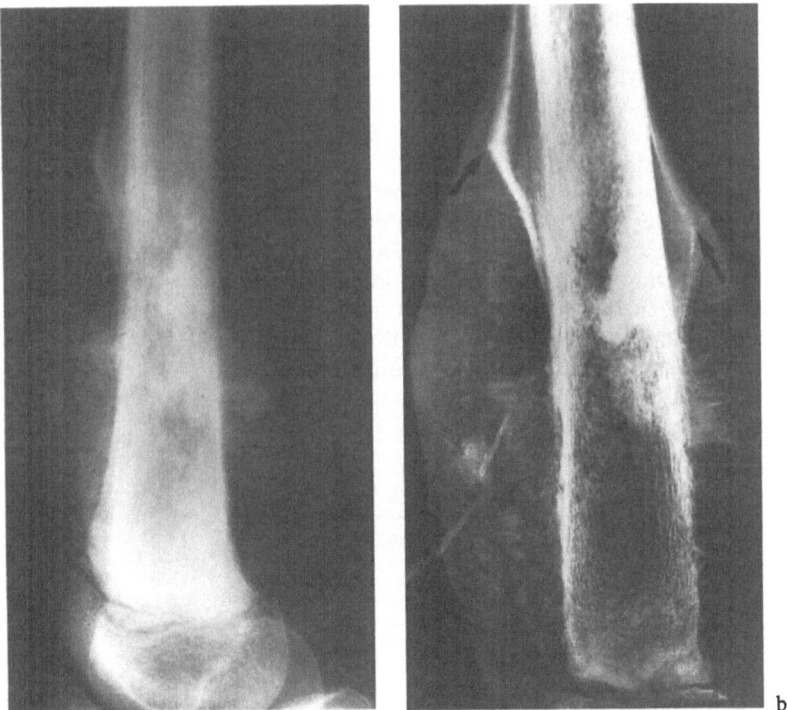

a   b

Fig. 5.12a,b. Perpendicular periosteal reaction and "Codman's triangle." Male, 13 years, osteogenic sarcoma of the femur. **a** In vivo, **b** specimen. There is a pronounced, perpendicularly oriented new bone formation, mainly along collagen fibers and vessels. Note the uplifted and interrupted periosteum in the proximal aspect of the cortical and periosteal breakthrough of tumor (*arrows*).

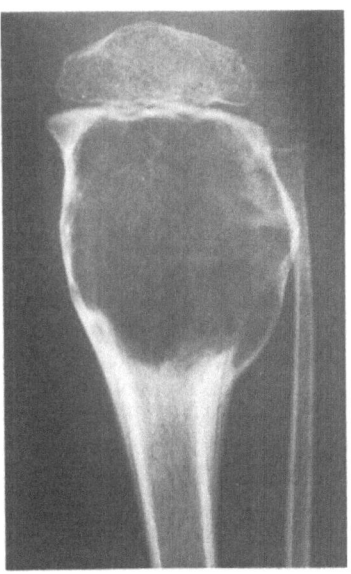

Fig. 5.13. Periosteal expanded shell. Male, 54 years, aneurysmal bone cyst.

A Simplified Classification of Local Behavior

Given the radiographic appearances of bone destruction and reaction, a classification into latent, active, and aggressive lesions can be made on the basis of the plain film radiograph (Table 5.2). The patterns of destruction and reaction in a given lesion are often mixed, and attention should be paid in the classification to the most aggressive signs: in an aggressive lesion there may be several areas with a "latent" or "active" appearance, but in a latent lesion there must be no changes consistent with active or aggressive tumors. Table 5.2 may give the impression that there are absolute and strict limits between latent, active, and aggressive lesions but, as stated earlier, there is a sliding scale from the very latent to the most aggressive patterns. Thus in some cases it may be difficult to place a lesion in one of two adjacent categories on the basis of radiographic findings only.

Table 5.2. Simplified radiographic classification of the local behavior of bone tumors

Local behavior	Radiologic characteristics
Latent	Geographic destruction
	Cortical "rim" or "capsule"
	Expanded cortex < 1 cm, if any
	Solid periosteal reaction, if any
Active	Geographic destruction
	Thin, well-defined transition zone
	Thin or no cortical capsule
	Cortical penetration acceptable
	Expanded cortex ≥ 1 cm
	Solid or lamellated periosteal reaction, if any
Aggressive	Moth-eaten/permeative destruction
	Ill-defined transition zone
	No cortical capsule
	Cortical and periosteal penetration
	Lamellated or perpendicular periosteal reaction
	Associated soft tissue mass

The Value of Other Modalities for Assessment of Local Behavior

In addition to plain film radiography, *scintigraphy* may give information on the aggressiveness of the tumor (Enneking 1983). In latent lesions scintigraphy with ^{99m}Tc-labelled phosphates or phosphonates usually reveals no significantly increased uptake, though there may be a thin zone of increased activity corresponding exactly to the mature reactive rim seen on the plain film radiograph (Fig. 5.14). In active lesions there is an increased uptake, corresponding in almost all cases to the area of involvement seen on the plain radiograph (Figs. 5.14 and 5.15). Aggressive lesions usually have considerably increased uptake, the area of which may extend well beyond the limits of the lesion as seen on the plain radiograph (Fig. 5.16). This "extended pattern of uptake" (Thrall et al. 1975) or "contiguous bone activity" (Simon and Kirchner 1980) will be discussed in Chapter 7. It should be noted that both active and aggressive lesions occasionally may have normal or even decreased uptake of the nucleotide (e.g. chordoma and myeloma).

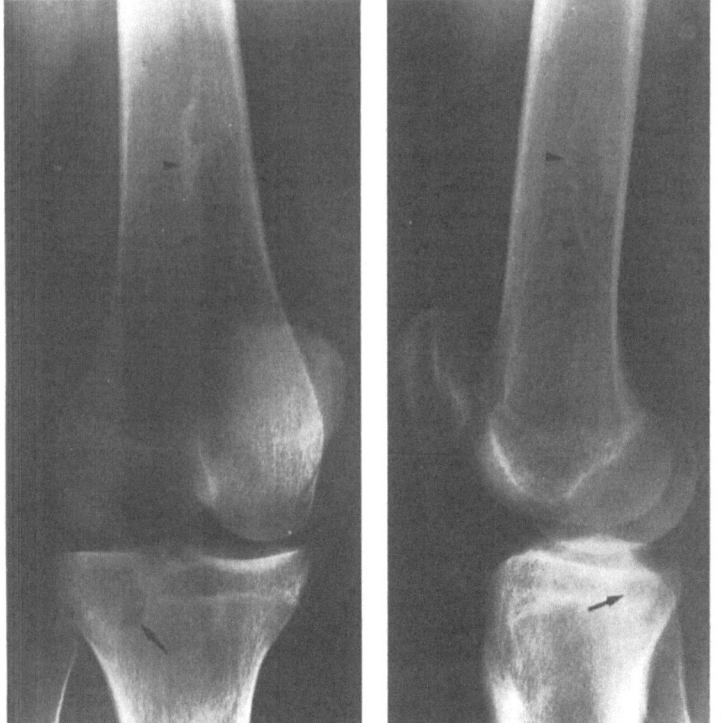

a   b

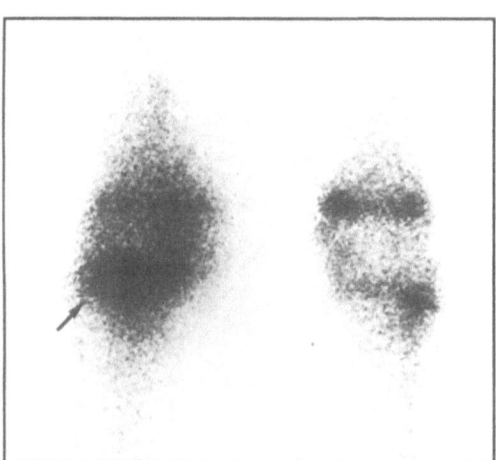

c

Fig. 5.14a–c. Latent and active lesions: plain film radiograph and scintigraphy. Female, 16 years, osteoblastoma of the proximal tibia and non-ossifying fibroma of the distal femur. **a** and **b** Plain film, anteroposterior and lateral projections. In the posterior part of the lateral tibial condyle there is osteolytic destruction with possible cortical breakthrough posteriorly (*arrow*). In the medial-posterior part of the distal femoral shaft there is a lesion with an appearance typical of a non-ossifying fibroma (*arrowheads*). **c** Scintigraphy. There is a generally increased uptake in the right knee, probably due to disuse osteopenia, and a pathologically increased uptake corresponding to the tibial lesion (*arrow*), consistent with an active lesion. The lesion in the distal femur has no or very faint increased uptake, consistent with a latent lesion.

As regards the concepts of malignant and benign, gallium-67 scans have been reported as 100% sensitive in depicting malignant bone tumors (Simon and Kirchner 1980), but are positive also in several benign tumors. At present neither ^{99m}Tc-labelled substances nor ^{67}Ga can be used to discriminate reliably between benign and malignant lesions (Silberstein 1984; Kirchner and Simon 1984).

Angiographic evaluation of the degree of malignancy of bone tumors has been thoroughly examined (Viamonte et al. 1973; Hudson et al. 1975, 1981; Levine et al. 1979). The classical radiologic signs of malignancy—neovascularity, arteriovenous shunts, vessel encasement, tumor blush—are reliable in most cases, provided that due consideration is given to changes caused by biopsy or fracture (Hudson et al. 1975). For intraosseous lesions, subtraction technique is strongly advisable since the bone texture will otherwise obscure the findings.

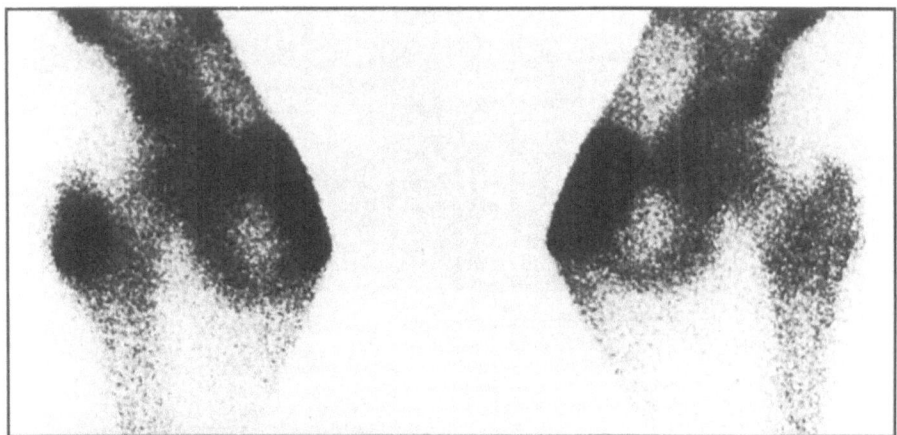

a

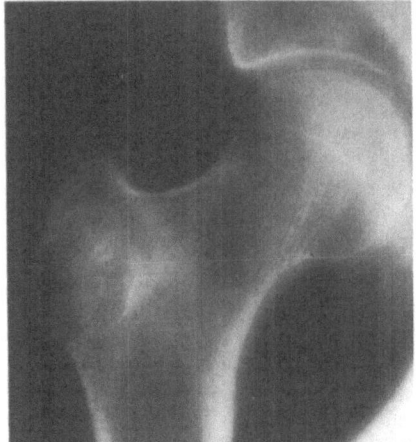

b

Fig. 5.15a,b. Active lesion: scintigraphy and conventional tomography. Female, 53 years, low-grade chondrosarcoma of the right greater trochanter. The area of increased uptake in the scintigram (a) corresponds well to the lesion as seen in a conventional tomogram (b).

With modern pharmacoangiography using tolazoline, epinephrine, angiotensin or prostanglandins, most authors report a rather direct correlation between the degree of pathologic vascularization and the dedifferentiation of tumors (Yaghmai et al. 1977; Levin et al. 1982), but angiographically avascular masses, although as a rule benign, may also be highly malignant. In accordance with Hudson et al. (1981), we have found arteriography to be of limited value in the assessment of the local behavior of bone tumors.

Computed tomography may reveal the destructive pattern of growth, especially in cancellous bone, more sensitively than plain films. Moreover, CT defines well the extension of tumor outside the bone (see Chapter 7), which is a sign of an aggressive tumor. Otherwise, CT is of limited value in the assessment of the aggressiveness of bone tumors.

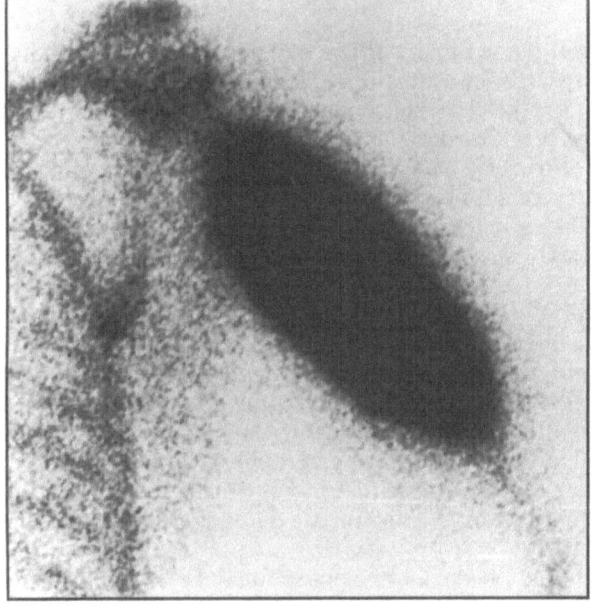
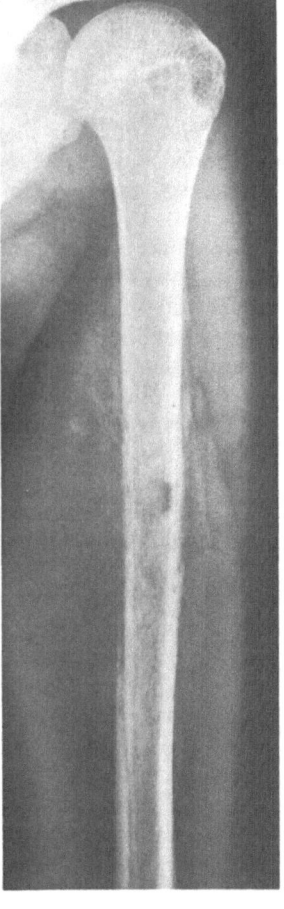

Fig. 5.16a,b. Aggressive lesion: scintigraphy and plain film radiography. Female, 16 years, osteogenic sarcoma of the humerus. The intensely increased uptake (**a**) extends beyond the lesion as seen at plain film examination (**b**).

In 1971, Damadian found increased T1 and T2 relaxation times in cancer specimens examined with nuclear magnetic resonance spectroscopy, and since then a large number of reports of increased relaxation times in malignant tissue based on spectroscopic examination in vitro have been published (Bottomley et al. 1984). Therefore, *magnetic resonance imaging* might have a potential for discriminating between malignant and benign tumors, by means of values of T1 and T2. However, in our experience (Pettersson et al. 1985) the relaxation times are increased to a varying degree in almost all musculoskeletal tumors (except lipomas) (Chapter 6). The degree of malignancy seems to have no impact on this. With present knowledge, therefore, relaxation times are of little value in the assessment of the aggressiveness of bone tumors.

Soft Tissue Tumors

The radiologic approach to soft tissue tumors differs in several respects from that to bone tumors, especially as regards the evaluation of local behavior.

If there is a bone reaction in the skeleton adjacent to the soft tissue tumor evident on the *plain film examination*, it is obvious that the tumor is locally aggressive, whether benign or malignant (Fig. 5.17). However, such a reaction is fairly seldom seen, and otherwise, plain film radiography has contributed little to the evaluation of the local behavior. Nevertheless, plain films should always be obtained to get an overview of the diseased area. They may also provide other important information for the radiologic work-up—for instance on the contents of the tumor matrix (calcification, fat, etc.)—as will be discussed in Chapter 6.

As with bone tumors, the *angiographic evaluation* may reveal dislocated vessels around a latent tumor and an increased vascularity both in the reactive margin and within the matrix of an aggressive tumor. However, the absence of increased vascularity is not a certain sign that the lesion is latent. Concerning the concepts benign and malignant, several authors advocate angiography as an important tool for determining the malignancy of a soft tissue tumor, but others do not (Hudson et al. 1975; Voegeli and Uehlinger 1976). We seldom use this method for the assessment of local behavior.

Scintigraphy with ^{99m}Tc-labelled phosphates or phosphonates is relatively inaccurate in the assessment of local aggressiveness. In the literature, a great deal of energy has been expended on the possibility of using scintigraphy to differentiate between benign and malignant tumors, while little attention has been focused on the local behavior (Enneking et al. 1981). Most malignant tumors exhibit increased uptake, and patients with benign tumors such as lipomas often have a normal scan (Chew and Hudson 1980). Thus, if a soft tissue lesion has no intrinsic uptake in the tumor and no increased uptake in the adjacent bone, it may safely be regarded as benign; it is also likely, but less certain, that it is latent (Chew et al. 1981). Increased intrinsic uptake is much less specific: it has been found in most malignant soft tissue tumors (Fig. 5.18), but also in several benign tumors, both active and latent (Fig. 5.18), and the findings are inconsistent (Chew and Hudson 1980; Chew et al. 1981).

Gallium-67 scans may be a more reliable preoperative indicator of malignant disease of soft tissue (Kaufmann et al. 1977; Bitran et al. 1978; Kirchner and Simon

1984). Kirchner and Simon (1981) found the combination of a positive gallium-67 scan and positive blood-pool images after injection of ^{99m}Tc-phosphonates to be a reasonably good indicator of the presence of a malignant soft tissue lesion; they achieved a sensitivity of 85% and a specificity of 92%. But the results reported by different authors are again inconsistent and partially contradictory (Lepanto et al. 1976; Kaufmann et al. 1977; Bitran et al. 1978; Teates et al. 1978; Zazzaro et al. 1980; Chew et al. 1981; Kirchner and Simon 1981).

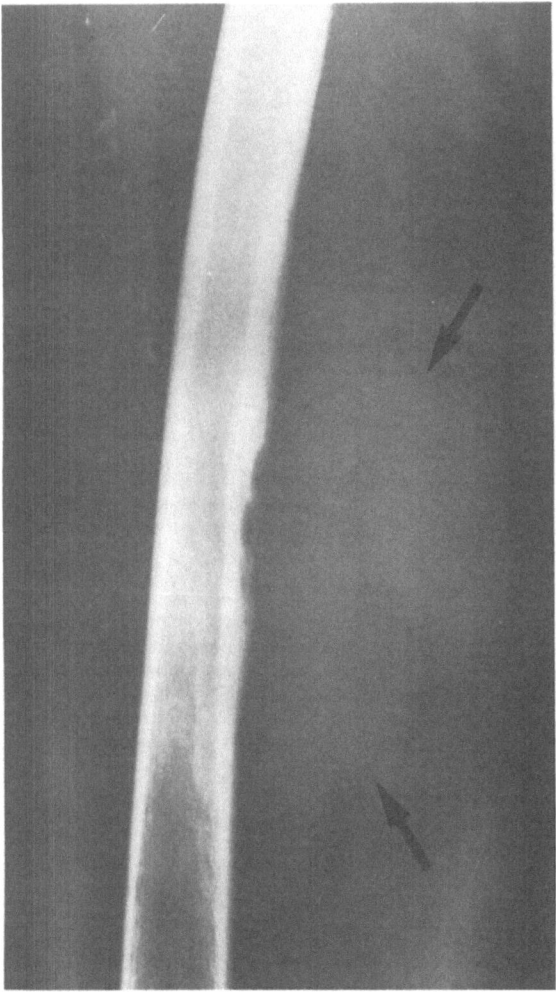

Fig. 5.17. Aggressive soft tissue tumor: plain film examination. Male, 72 years, fibrosarcoma of the posterior thigh. There is a large soft tissue tumor (*arrows*) with destruction of the outer aspect of the femoral cortex.

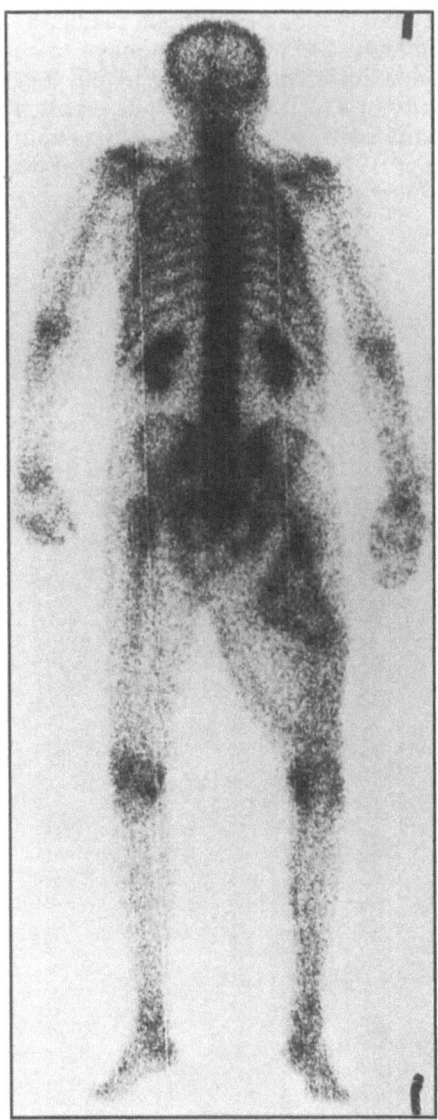

Fig. 5.18. Liposarcoma of the thigh with one sarcomatous and one lipomatous portion: scintigraphy. Male, 73 years. Posterior view. The right thigh is considerably increased in size, and there is a triangular area with increased uptake. Only this part contained malignant tissue.

With *computed tomography* and *magnetic resonance imaging* the diagnosis of a lipoma can be made with certainty, as will be described in Chapter 6. Given this diagnosis the lesion may safely be regarded as benign. Otherwise, these modalities contribute no additional information as to the aggressiveness. Therefore, unless the diagnosis of a lipoma is made, all deep soft tissue tumors should be approached as though they were aggressive (Springfield et al. 1984).

References

Bitran JD, Bekerman C, Golomb HM, Simon MA (1978) Scintigraphic evaluation of sarcomata in children and adults by Ga[67] citrate. Cancer 42: 1760–1765

Bottomley PA, Foster TH, Argensinger RE, Pfefier LM (1984) A review of normal tissue hydrogen NMR relaxation times and relaxation mechanisms from 1–100 MHz: Dependence on tissue type, NMR frequency, temperature, species, excision and age. Review article. Med Phys 11: 425–447

Brunschwig A, Harmon PH (1935) Studies in bone sarcoma. III. An experimental and pathological study of the role of the periosteum in the formation of bone in various primary bone tumors. Surg Gynecol Obstet 60: 30–40

Chew FS, Hudson TM (1980) Radionuclide imaging of lipoma and liposarcoma. Radiology 136: 741–745

Chew FS, Hudson TM, Enneking WF (1981) Radionuclide imaging of soft tissue neoplasms. Semin Nucl Med 11: 266–276

Damadian RV (1971) Tumor detection by nuclear magnetic resonance. Science 171: 1151–1153

Edeiken J (1981) Roentgen diagnosis of diseases of bone, 3rd edn. Williams and Wilkins, Baltimore, pp 11–29

Edeiken J, Hodes PJ, Caplan LH (1966) New bone production and periosteal reaction. AJR 97: 708–718

Enneking WF (1977) Clinical musculoskeletal pathology. Storter Printing Company, Gainesville, Florida, pp 1–33

Enneking WF (1983) Musculoskeletal tumor surgery. Churchill Livingstone, Edinburgh, pp 141–168

Enneking WF, Chew FS, Springfield DS, Hudson TM, Spanier SS (1981) The role of radionuclide bone-scanning in determining the resectability of soft-tissue sarcomas. J Bone Joint Surg [Am] 63: 249–257

Garber CZ (1951) Reactive bone formation in Ewing's sarcoma. Cancer 4: 839–845

Hudson TM, Haas G, Enneking WF, Hawkins JR (1975) Angiography in the management of musculoskeletal tumors. Surg Gynecol Obstet 141: 11–21

Hudson TM, Enneking WF, Hawkins JF (1981) The value of angiography in planning surgical treatment of bone tumors. Radiology 138: 283–292

Kaufmann JH, Cedermark BJ, Parthasarathy KL, Didolkar MS, Bakshi SP (1977) The value of ^{67}Ga scintigraphy in soft tissue sarcoma and chondrosarcoma. Radiology 123: 131–134

Kirchner PT, Simon MA (1981) Current concepts review. Radioisotopic evaluation of skeletal disease. J Bone Joint Surg [Am] 63: 673–681

Kirchner PT, Simon MA (1984) The clinical value of bone and gallium scintigraphy for soft-tissue sarcomas of the extremities. J Bone Joint Surg [Am] 66: 319–327

Kricun ME (1983) Radiographic evaluation of solitary bone lesions. Orth Clin North Am 14: 39–64

Lepanto PB, Rosenstock J, Littman P, Alavi A, Donaldson M, Kuhl DE (1976) Gallium-67 scans in children with solid tumors. AJR 126: 179–186

Levin DC, Watson RC, Ballaie HA (1982) Arteriography in diagnosis and management of acquired peripheral soft tissue masses. Radiology 103: 53–58

Levine E, Lee KR, Neff JR, Mahlad F, Robinson RG, Preston DF (1979) Comparison of computed tomography and other imaging modalities in the evaluation of musculoskeletal tumors. Radiology 131: 431–437

Lodwick GS (1966a) Computer aided diagnosis in radiology: A research plan. Invest Radiol 1: 72–80

Lodwick GS (1966b) Solitary malignant tumors of bone: The application of predictor variables in diagnosis. Semin Roentgenol 1: 293–313

Lodwick GS (1971) Atlas of tumor radiology. The bones and joints. Year Book Medical Publishers, Chicago, pp 65–79

Lodwick GS, Wilson AJ, Farrell C, Virtama P, Dittrich F (1980a) Determining growth rates of focal lesions of bone from radiographs. Radiology 134: 577–583

Lodwick GS, Wilson AJ, Farrell C, Virtama P, Smeltzer FM, Dittrich F (1980b) Estimating rate of growth in bone lesions: Observer performance and error. Radiology 134: 585–590

Madewell JE, Ragsdale BD, Sweet DE (1981) Radiologic and pathologic analysis of solitary bone lesions. I. Internal margins. Radiol Clin North Am 19: 715–748

Nelson SW (1966) Some fundamentals in the radiologic differential diagnosis of solitary bone lesions. Semin Roentgenol 1: 244–266

Norman A, Ulin R (1969) A comparative study of periosteal new-bone response in metastatic bone tumors (solitary) and primary bone sarcomas. Radiology 92: 705–708

Pettersson H, Spanier S, Fitzsimmons JR, Slone R, Scott KN (1985) MR imaging relaxation measurements in musculoskeletal tumors and surrounding tissue. Radiology 157(P): 109

Ragsdale BD, Madewell JE, Sweet DE (1981) Radiologic and pathologic analysis of solitary bone lesions. II. Periosteal reactions. Radiol Clin North Am 19: 749–783

Rosenthal DJ, Schiller AL, Mankin HJ (1984) Chondrosarcoma: Correlation of radiological and histological grade. Radiology 150: 21–26

Silberstein EB (1984) Bone scintigraphy. Futura Publishing Company, New York, pp 259–277

Simon MA, Kirchner PT (1980) Scintigraphic evaluation of primary bone tumors. J Bone Joint Surg [Am] 62: 758–764

Springfield DS, Enneking WF, Neff JR, Mahley JT (1984) Principles of tumor management. In: Murray JA (ed) AAOS Instructional Course Lectures. CV Mosby, St. Louis, pp 1–25

Teates CD, Bray ST, Williamson BRJ (1978) Tumor detection with ^{67}Ga citrate: A literature survey (1970–1978). Clin Nucl Med 3: 456–460

Thrall JH, Geslien GE, Corcoron RJ, Johnson MC (1975) Abnormal radionuclide deposition patterns adjacent to focal skeletal lesions. Radiology 115: 659–663

Viamonte M, Roen S, Lepage J (1973) Nonspecificity of abnormal vascularity in the angiographic diagnosis of malignant neoplasms. Radiology 106: 59–67

Voegeli E, Uehlinger E (1976) Arteriography in bone tumors. Skeletal Radiol 1: 3–14

Wilner D (1982) Radiology of bone tumors and allied disorders. WB Saunders, Philadelphia, pp 25–75

Yaghmai J, Zia A, Shariat S et al. (1971) Value of arteriography in the diagnosis of benign and malignant bone lesions. Cancer 27: 1134–1147

Zazzaro PF, Bosworth JE, Schneider V, Zelenak JJ (1980) Gallium scanning in malignant fibrous histocytoma. AJR 135: 775–779

Chapter 6
Radiologic Diagnosis

The diagnostic classification of a musculoskeletal tumor is based upon histogenic patterns and should be made by the pathologist only with thorough knowledge of the radiologic and clinical data. But in many bone lesions a nearly certain diagnosis can be made on the basis of the radiologic findings alone. This radiologic diagnosis, even when not definitive, is important for the planning of the future management of the patient (Springfield et al. 1984).

In the radiologic diagnostic work-up a systematic approach is very useful and should involve analysis of several parameters:

1. Age of the patient and pertinent clinical information (pain, growth rate and size of a palpable mass, heat, tenderness, mobility, laboratory data etc.)
2. Singularity or multiplicity of the tumor
3. Localization in the body and in the bone
4. Size and shape of the tumor
5. Specific radiologic patterns of the tumor matrix
6. Local behavior of the tumor

These parameters will be discussed briefly below, except for the local behavior which has been dealt with in the previous chapter; however, only the principles will be discussed, with primary emphasis being laid on the impact of the different imaging modalities.

The radiographic characteristics of bone tumors have been thoroughly studied over a period of many decades, and are the subject of several extensive texts (Dahlin 1978; Wilner 1982; Edeiken 1983; Hudson 1986). For detailed information concerning the diagnostic classification of a lesion in an individual patient, such texts should be consulted; it is far beyond the scope of this book to discuss details of the individual tumors.

Age of the Patient and Pertinent Clinical Information

The age of the patient is of great importance in the diagnosis. The age prevalence is well documented for the primary bone tumors (Table 6.1). For detailed information on the age distribution of the different tumors the reader is referred to current texts.

Not only the patient's age, but the entire the clinical history, including the duration of symptoms, hereditary background and laboratory data should also be considered before the radiologic diagnosis is made.

Table 6.1. Some variables of solitary bone lesions (from Kricun 1983, with permission)

	Pattern destr.[a]	Rate of growth[b]					Matrix[c]	Periosteal reaction	Age (decades)	Location in long bones[d]	Reactive bone	Total blastic	Mult. lesions	Other
		1A	1B	1C	2	3								
Benign														
Aneurysmal bone cyst	G	●	+	+	●		—	Lamellated (occ.)	1–3	Any	Margin (rare)	—	—	Expansile; ¾ under 20 years old
Chondroblastoma	G	+	+	+	●		Ca^{2+}, punctate	Lamellated (occ.)	2, 3	M E	Margin	—	—	25% calcify. Epiphysis. ¾ under 20
Chondromyxoid fibroma	G	+	+	+			Ca^{2+}, punctate	—	2, 3	M	Margin	—	—	May grow to cartilage plate. 2% calcify. Rare
Cyst	G	+	+				—	—	1, 2	M D	Margin	—	—	Central. Floating fragment. Proximal humerus, proximal femur
Enchondroma	G	+	+				Ca^{2+}; punctate, arcs, rings	—	2–5	M	Margin	—	+	Hands, long bones. Frequent calcification
Fibrous dysplasia	G	+	+				Osteoid; Ca^{2+}, punctate	—	1–3	D m	Margin	Occ.	+ +	Central, elongated. May ossify or calcify
Giant cell tumor	G	●	+	+			—	—	3, 4	M–E	Margin (rare)	—	—	Frequent expansion. 90% over 20. Grows into epiphysis
Histiocytosis	GMP	+	+	+	+	●	—	Solid, sing. layer, mult. layer (rare)	1–3	D m	Margin	—	+ +	Beveled edge. 70% solitary
Non-ossifying fibroma	G	+	●				Osteoid (late)	—	1–3	M	Margin	Occ.	+	Cortical; scalloped. Metadiaphysis. Frequent
Osteoblastoma	G	+	+	●			Osteoid; Ca^{2+}, punctate	—	2, 3	M	Margin	Occ.	—	Posterior spine, long bones, hands
Osteochondroma	—		●				Ca^{2+} punctate, arcs, rings	—	2, 3	M	—	—	+	Cartilage cap may calcify. Points away from joint
Osteoid osteoma	G	+	●				—	Solid, layer (occ.)	2, 3	D m	Intense	+ +	—	Reaction greater than lesion. Nidus
Osteomyelitis	GMP	+	●	●	●	+	Sequestrum	Solid, sing. layer, mult. layer	Any 1	M d	Margin, mottled	Occ.	+ (occ.)	Destroys cartilage; sequestrum; sinus tract; involucrum

	Pattern destr.[a]	Rate of growth[b]					Matrix[c]	Periosteal reaction	Age (decades)	Location in long bones[d]	Reactive bone	Total blastic	Mult. lesions	Other
		1A	1B	1C	2	3								
Malignant														
Adamantinoma	G	+	+	+	●		Ca²⁺ (occ.), punctate	—	2–4	D	Margin	—	—	Mid and distal third tibia. Rare
Chondrosarcoma	G p	+	+	+	+	+	Ca²⁺; punctate, arcs, rings	Velvet (occ.)	4–6	M d	—	—	—	Pelvis, flat bones, proximal femur; all calcify
Chordoma	G		+	+			Ca²⁺, punctate	—	4–7	—	Margin	—	—	Sacrum, clivus, C-spine. Presacral mass
Ewing's sarcoma	P				●	+	—	Sing. or multi. layer, hair-on-end	1–3	D M	Mottled, intense (occ.)	Occ.	—	Saucerization
Fibrosarcoma	G p	●	+	+	+		—	Amorphous (occ.)	2–6	M	—	—	—	—
Giant cell tumor	G	●	+	+			—	—	3–6	M–E	Margin (occ.)	—	—	Frequent expansion. Grows into epiphysis
Histiocytic lymphoma (reticulum cell sarcoma)	M p			●	+		—	Amorphous	3–6	D M	Mottled	—	+ +	—
Metastasis	G M P	●	+	+	+	+	—	Sing. layer, sunburst, hair-on-end, solid (rare)	Any 5 +	M D e	Margin (occ.)	+ + +	+ + + +	Saucerization; red marrow; most frequent destructive lesion 40 +
Myeloma	G p	●	+	+	●		—	—	5 +	M D	—	Rare	+ + + +	Red marrow. Most frequent primary bone tumor
Osteosarcoma	P g			●	+	+	+ Tumor bone	Sunburst, hair-on-end, mult., sing. layer	2, 3, 6	M d	—	+ +	+ Rare	Most frequent primary bone tumor after myeloma
Parosteal sarcoma	—					●	Tumor bone	—	3, 4	M d	—	+ + +	—	Cleavage plane

[a] Upper case letters denote frequent, lower case letters denote less frequent. G, geographic; M, moth-eaten; P, permeated.
[b] Adapted from Lodwick. +, frequent; ●, frequent; , less frequent. [c] Ca²⁺, calcification; occ., occasional.
[d] Upper case letters denote frequent, lower case letters denote less frequent. D, diaphysis; E, epiphysis; M, metaphysis.

Singularity or Multiplicity of the Tumor

In the evaluation of *bone tumors*, screening for multiple lesions in the body is a very useful first step, since the presence of such lesions will totally change the approach to treatment. The best modality in this respect is a scintigraphic whole body survey using ⁹⁹mTc-labelled phosphates or phosphonates (Kirchner and Simon 1984). Bone scintigraphy will reveal such frequently multiple focal lesions as enchondroma, osteochondroma and histiocytosis X, as well as metastatic cancer (Blair and McAfee 1976; Citrin et al. 1977). It will also uncover, for instance, multifocal osteosarcoma and metastases from osteogenic or Ewing's sarcoma (Gilday et al. 1977; McNeil 1978) (Fig. 6.1).

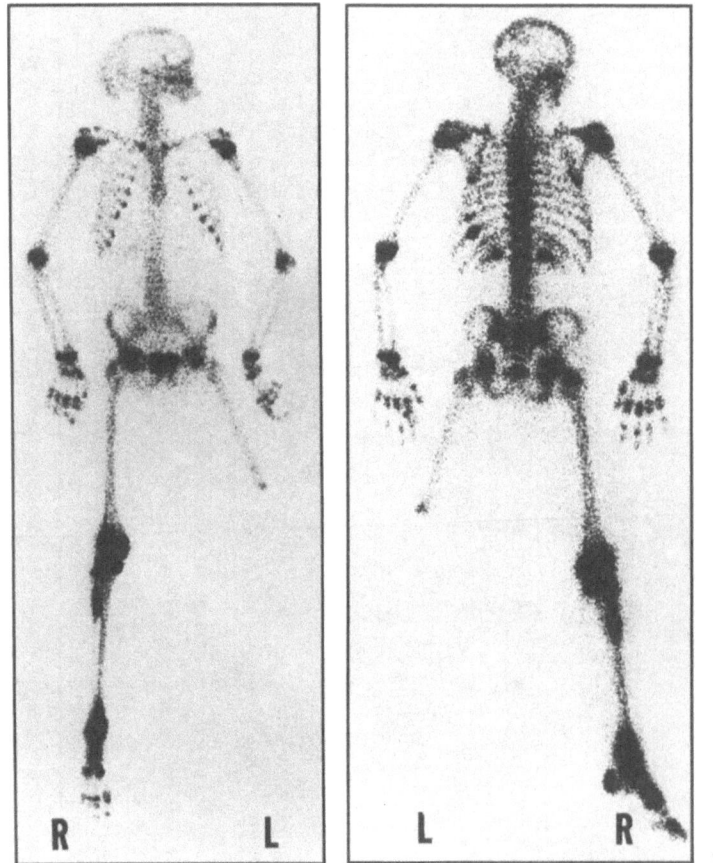

Fig. 6.1a,b. Multiple skeletal metastases: scintigraphy. Male, 11 years, 9 months after above-knee amputation of the left leg because of osteosarcoma of the proximal tibia. **a** Anterior and **b** posterior view. R, right; L, left. There are areas with increased uptake caused by metastases in the ninth and tenth left ribs, the right greater trochanter, the proximal right fibula and the distal right tibia. The increased uptake in the distal end of the left femur is caused by remodelling at the amputation site.

Before the era of modern chemotherapy, skeletal metastases from osteosarcomas were seldom found prior to metastases to the lung and were seen in only 1%–2% of patients when the primary tumor was diagnosed (Goldstein et al. 1980; McKillop et al. 1981). Today, during and after chemotherapy, bone metastases are much more frequently seen prior to lung metastases, and may appear as the first sign of spread of the malignancy in up to 16% of patients who develop generalized disease (Goldstein et al. 1980).

"Skip lesions", i.e. local metastases to the skeleton (Enneking and Kagan 1975), or multiple primary tumors in the neighborhood of the one initially discovered may also be detected by bone scintigraphy (Enneking and Kagan 1975; Enneking 1983) (Fig. 6.2). CT and MRI have been reported to be of value too in such cases (Pettersson et al. 1985c) (Fig. 6.3).

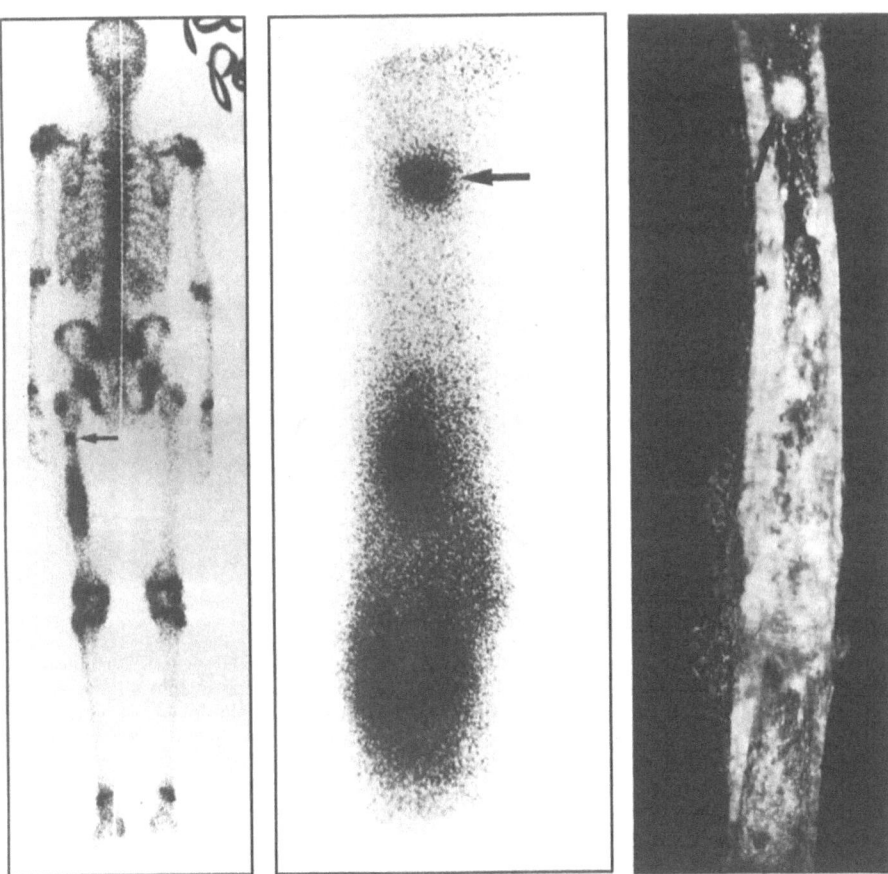

a   b,c

Fig. 6.2a–c. Skip lesion: scintigraphy. Male, 14 years, osteogenic sarcoma. **a** The whole body scintigram and **b** the spot film show increased uptake in the shaft of the femur, caused by the primary tumor. Proximal to this there is a small area of increased uptake (*arrow*), consistent with a skip lesion. **c** Specimen, under ultraviolet light for tetracycline fluoroscence. The primary tumor and the skip lesion (*arrow*) are well visualized.

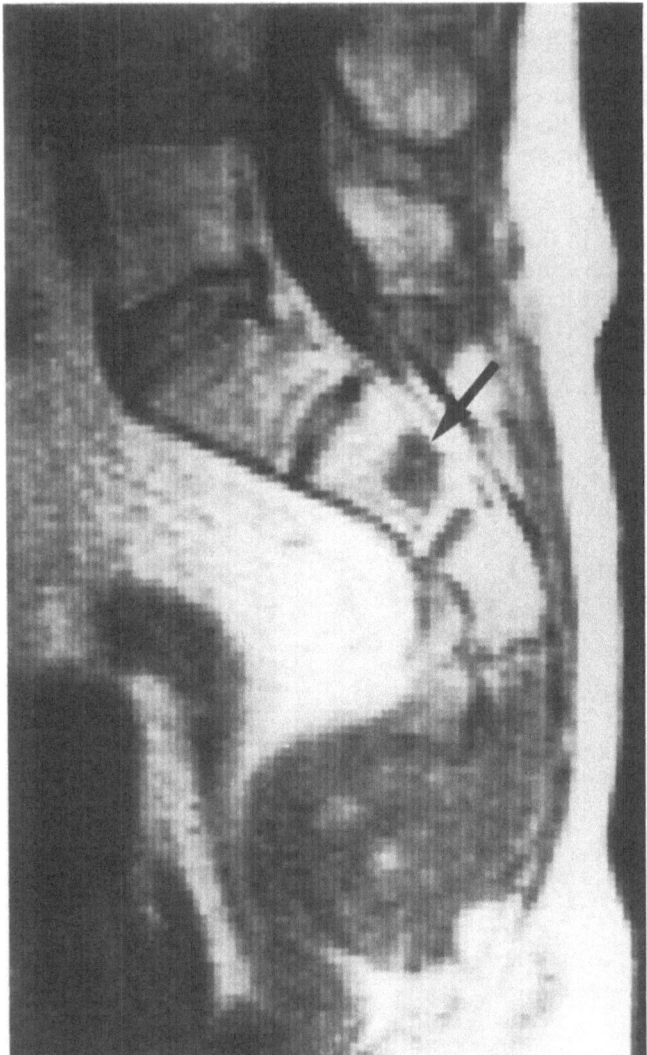

Fig. 6.3. Skip lesion: MRI. Male, 59 years, chordoma. SE 500/30 ms. In the sagittal plane the lesion extending from vertebral bodies S4–S5 is obvious. In the S2 vertebral body there is a lesion (*arrow*) with the same signal intensity as the large lesion. Both lesions proved to be chordoma.

It should be noted, however, that not all bone tumors have an increased uptake at scinitigraphy. Thus, in some cases of eosinophilic granuloma, in patients with anaplastic metastases and, especially, in suspected myeloma, a plain film skeletal survey is recommended.

If a potentially malignant primary bone or soft tissue tumor is diagnosed, a plain film chest examination should routinely be performed in the seach for lung metastases. To the routine anteroposterior (AP) and lateral views, an "over-penetrated" AP view may be added. This will minimize the risk of overlooking

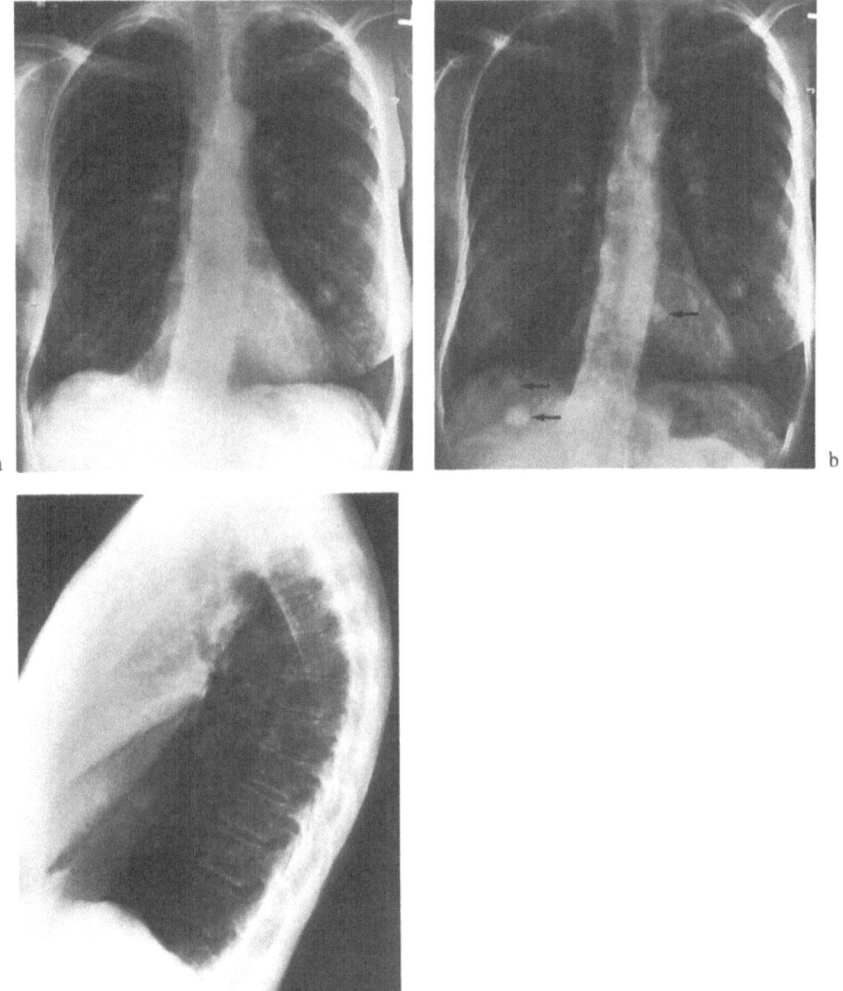

Fig. 6.4a–c. Lung metastases: plain film chest examination. Female, 72 years, chondrosarcoma of the left scapula. Status 14 months after marginal excision. **a** AP, normal exposure. **b** AP, "overpenetrated." **c** Lateral view. The patient could not raise her left arm.

There are multiple metastases in both lungs. In the overpenetrated view (**b**) the lesions in the dorsal right phrenicocostal sinus and in the left paraspinal region (*arrows*) are more clearly seen than on the normally exposed film. Note the possible breakthrough of the primary tumor into the thoracic cavity (*arrowhead*).

metastases, especially near the mediastinum and in the phrenicocostal sinuses (Fig. 6.4), partly because of the different exposures and partly because the radiologist may then interpret two AP projections that are not identical with respect to respiration: a small metastasis that may be obscured behind a vessel or rib on one view may be visible on the other view. An alternative routine would be to add two oblique views to the AP and lateral. Lung metastases from osteogenic sarcoma or other bone-forming tumors may also be detected by scintigraphy (Fig. 6.5).

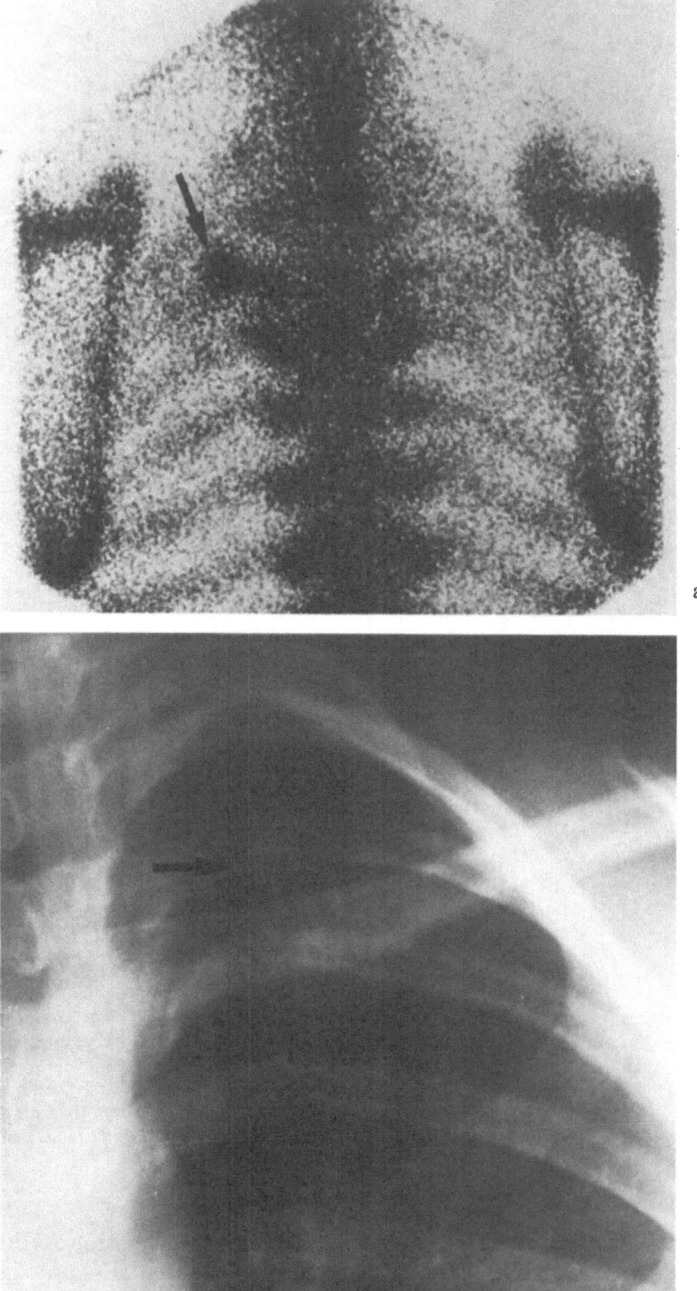

Fig. 6.5a,b. Lung metastasis: scintigraphy and plain film. Same patient as Fig. 6.1, 3 years later. The skeletal metastases had been successfully treated with chemotherapy. **a** Scintigram, posterior view. There is an area of increased uptake between the second and third left ribs, consistent with lung metastasis (*arrow*). **b** Plain film, showing the metastasis in the left upper lobe (*arrow*).

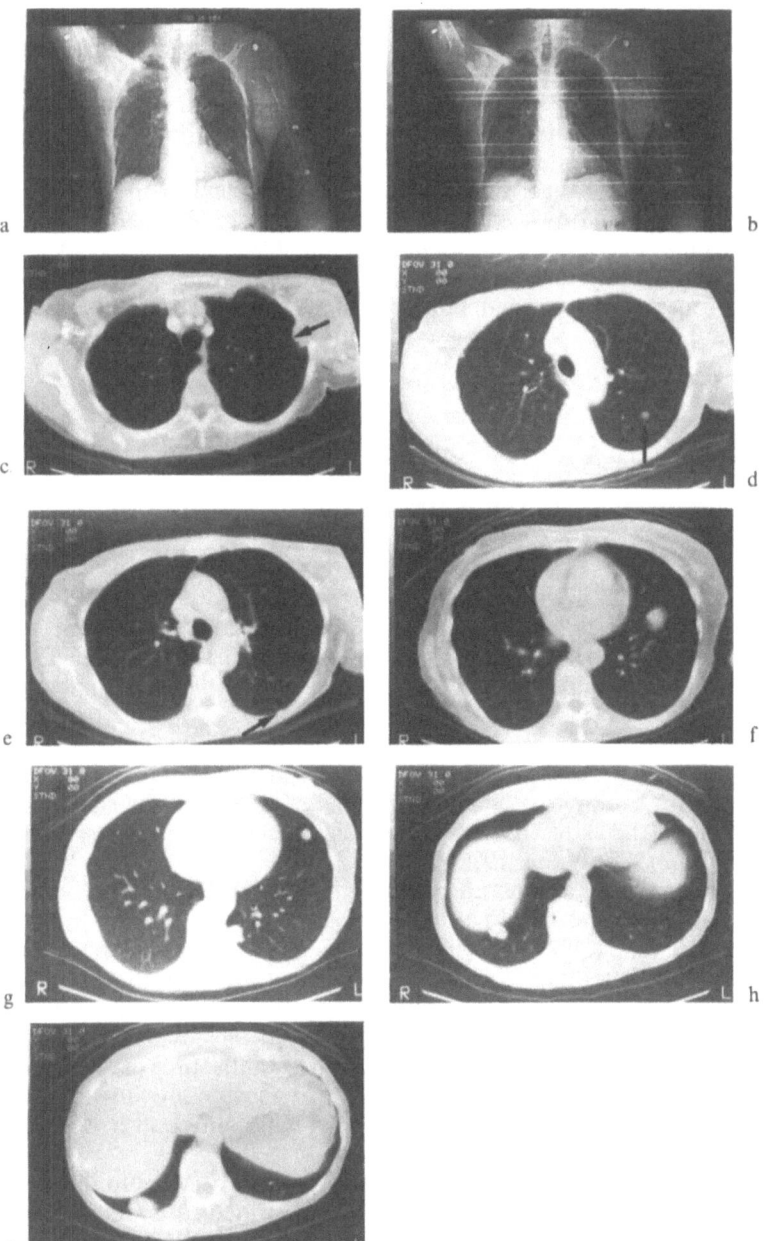

Fig. 6.6a–i. Lung metastases: CT. Same patient and occasion as Fig. 6.3. **a** and **b** Digital radiograph without and with selective sections outlined. **c–i** The sections as outline in **b**.

Most of the metastases revealed at the CT examination were seen also at the plain film examinations (compare Fig. 6.4), but the small lesions seen in sections 10 and 11 (**d,e**; *arrows*) are not visible on the plain films, not even retrospectively. The breakthrough of the primary tumor into the thoracic cavity is obvious (**c**; *arrow*).

Today the most sensitive and specific modality for the detection of lung metastases is CT, and we recommend a chest CT as a baseline examination before surgery for all patients with musculoskeletal tumors that may be malignant. In the follow-up controls plain film examination should be sufficient as a routine evaluation of lung metastases, and CT should again be performed if the chest film is inconclusive or if metastases are detected and surgery considered (Fig. 6.6).

For *soft tissue tumors* a thorough clinical examination is crucial, both for detection of the primary tumor and for evaluation of its multiplicity (Springfield et al. 1984). CT and MRI may also add important information due to their high contrast resolution of soft tissue (Pettersson et al. 1985a,c). Scintigraphy plays a relatively minor role in this respect, but its potential for detecting soft tissue tumors has been stressed by some authors.

Localization in the Body and in the Bone

Most *bone tumors* may occur anywhere in the skeleton, but several tumor groups exhibit a predilection for certain sites. As described above, bone scintigraphy is the most suitable method for detecting which part or parts of the skeleton are affected, while the plain film examination will reveal the localization within the bone in more detail.

The type of bone involved may be important. Most primary bone tumors appear in the large long bones, while some others tend to affect the flat bones, small long bones, or vertebrae: for example, osteoma in the skull, angioma in the skull and vertebrae, chordoma in the skull base or sacrum, and enchondroma in the hand (Mangini 1967; Dahlin 1978; Wilner 1982).

Within the long bones the areas most affected are the sites of rapid growth: proximal humerus, distal femur and proximal tibia. According to the metabolic field theory of Johnson (1953), a tumor of a given cell type most often develops in the metabolic field where the homologous normal cells are most active. In concordance with this, most tumors develop in the metaphysis. But again there are several exceptions: chondroblastoma often occurs in the epiphysis before closure of the physis, and a giant cell tumor most often extends into the epiphysis at the time of diagnosis (Kricun 1983). Round cell tumor and adamantinoma most often involve the diaphysis. Within the flat bones the localization is less specific, and can very seldom be used for diagnostic purposes (Wilner 1982).

The symmetrical or asymmetrical positioning of a tumor in relation to the axis of a long bone may give additional information. Many primary tumors arise in the medullary cavity, but most are, as a rule, asymmetrically positioned (e.g. giant cell tumor and chondroblastoma), and only a few are symmetric (such as chordoma) (Wilner 1982). Tumors arising in the cortical bone, such as osteoid osteoma, ossifying and non-ossifying fibroma, and tumors arising juxtacortically, such as osteochondroma, periosteal and parosteal osteosarcoma, are by definition asymmetrically placed. However, most other tumors, such as osteosarcoma, chondrosarcoma and fibrosarcoma, may be either symmetric or asymmetric, and the symmetry of the tumor is therefore of limited diagnostic value.

As to the localization of *soft tissue tumors*, CT and MRI will reveal the position most accurately (Rosenthal 1982, 1985; Pettersson et al. 1985c; Zimmer et al. 1985). However, this is more important for the surgical planning than for the diagnosis and will be discussed in the following chapter.

Size and Shape of the Tumor

The size and shape of *bone tumors* as evaluated at the plain film examination may add some information of relevance to the diagnosis. A malignant tumor is generally larger than 6 cm in diameter and often more than 9 cm at diagnosis (Lodwick 1971). Benign tumors are usually less than 6 cm and often less then 3 cm. Benign tumors tend to grow circumferentially while malignant tumors may grow in any direction (Wilner 1982). The variation within each tumor group is large, however, and only occasionally will the size and shape contribute significantly to the diagnosis.

The size and shape of *soft tissue tumors* vary considerably at diagnosis, depending upon position and possible concomitant symptoms, and have little correlation with the diagnosis.

Specific Radiologic Patterns of the Tumor Matrix

The pattern of the tumor matrix as revealed by the different diagnostic modalities may be of value in the diagnosis, but often the pattern is non-specific. The information available varies considerably between the modalities.

Plain Film Radiography

Many primary *bone tumors* do not produce any matrix that is visible on the plain film, and will thus appear radiolucent. Other tumors may produce mineralized tissue, visible on the plain film as calcification or ossification. For instance, in fibrous dysplasia, osteoblastoma and occasionally osteosarcoma, there may be numerous very small mineral deposits causing a diffusely increased density, the so-called ground glass appearance (Fig. 6.7a) (Hudson 1986).

Osteosarcomas often form abnormal new tumor bone that is visible as irregular or dense solid areas (Figs. 6.7b and 7.2), and especially when this occurs in tumor extending into the soft tissue it may appear as amorphous "cloudy" lesions (Fig. 6.7a).

In most enchondromas and chondrosarcomas, occasionally in chondroblastomas, and rarely in chondromyxoid fibromas, some calcifications are punctuated and/or ring-like (Feldman et al. 1970; McLeod and Beabout 1973; Sweet et al. 1981; Zlatkin et al. 1985). They may appear as whole rings, described by several authors as "smoke rings", or as broken rings or "arcs" (Fig. 6.8) (Feldman et al. 1970; McLeod and Beabout 1973; Enneking 1977; Sweet et al. 1981; Zlatkin et al. 1985).

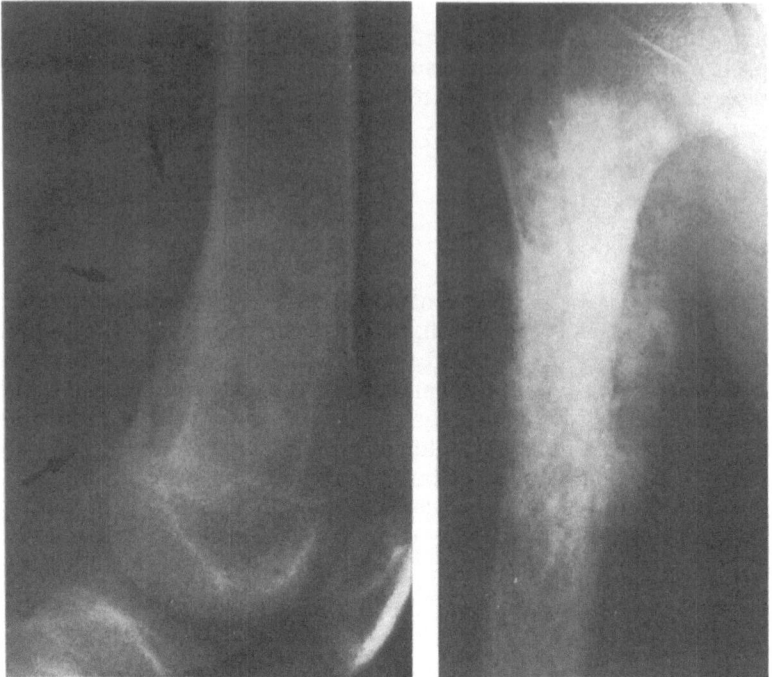

a   b

Fig. 6.7a,b. Different appearances of new bone formation. **a** Male, 15 years, osteogenic sarcoma. **b** Male, 18 years, osteogenic sarcoma. **a** The abnormal new bone may appear as a diffuse area of increased density ("ground glass appearance"). In the soft tissue the bone may look amorphous ("cloudy", *arrows*). **b** The tumor bone may appear irregular and dense, totally replacing the bone where it has arisen.

In *soft tissue tumors* plain film examinations give little diagnostic information. However, the low density of a lipoma can be appreciated (Fig. 6.9), as can the calcified phlebolites of a tumor of vascular origin (Fig. 4.1) (Hudson 1986). Calcifications may also be seen in synovial cell sarcoma. Xeroradiography, because of its broad latitude and edge enhancement, may reveal soft tissue tumors better than conventional plain films (Fig. 6.10) (Martel and Abell 1973; Bernardino et al. 1981). In general, however, plain film radiography and xeroradiography are non-specific for diagnosis of soft tissue tumors.

Ultrasound

In bone tumors, ultrasonography has so far been of no diagnostic use. New techniques with ultrasound of very high frequency may change this, but as yet no clinical experiences of such examinations have been reported.

In the evaluation of soft tissue tumors, ultrasound may be used to differentiate between solid and cystic lesions. Cystic lesions are non-echogenic, often with an increased echo behind the lesions (Pettersson et al. 1985b) (Fig. 6.11), while solid lesions give echos of mixed intensity (Fig. 6.12). Calcifications within the lesion

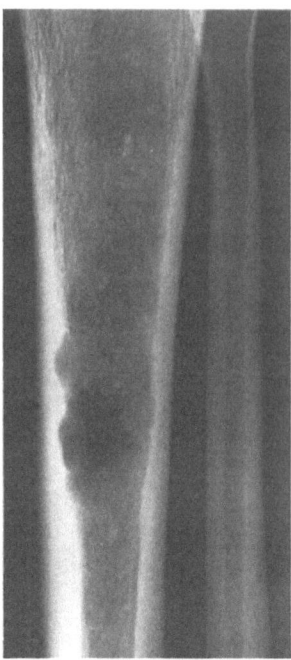

Fig. 6.8. Intraosseous calcification in a cartilaginous tumor. Female, 50 years, chondrosarcoma. The ossifications typically appear as "rings" or "arcs."

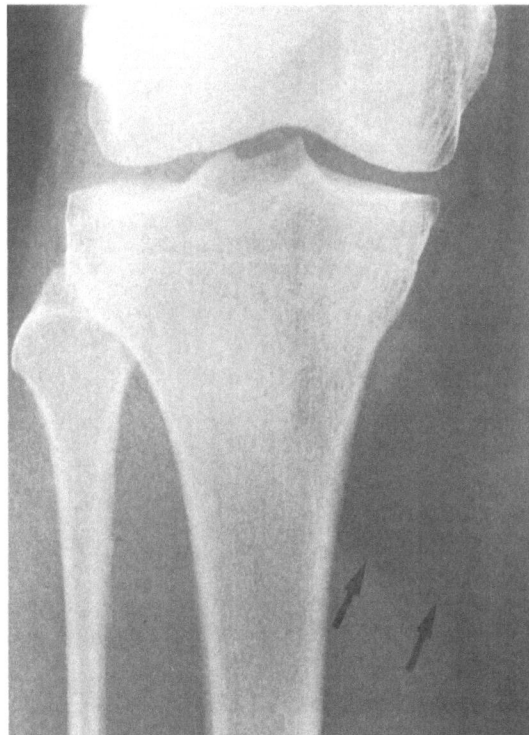

Fig. 6.9. Low-density lesion: plain film examination. Female, 60 years, lipoma. Such low density (*arrows*) is most often seen in lipomas and liposarcomas, but the findings are not diagnostic.

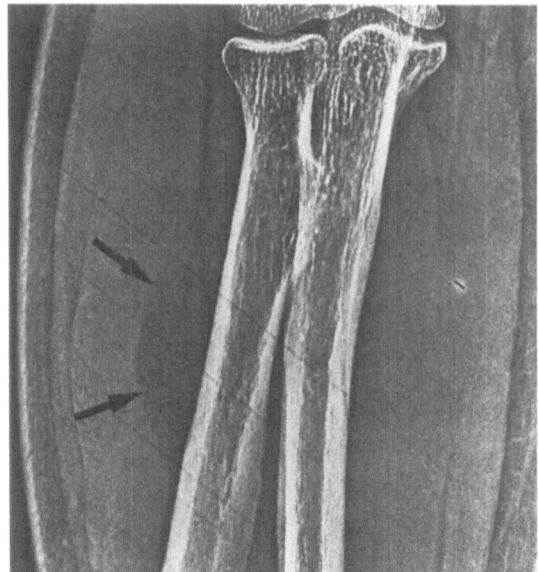

Fig. 6.10. Low-density lesion: xeroradiography. Female, 50 years, lipoma. The lesion (*arrows*) could barely be seen at plain film radiography.

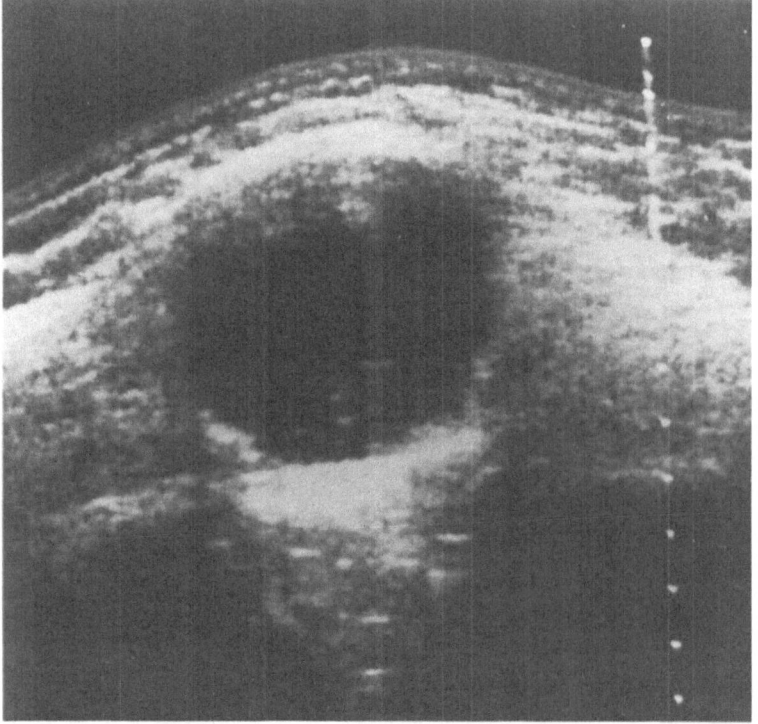

Fig. 6.11. Cystic tumor: ultrasound. Female, 43 years, cystic myxoma. There are no echos from the cystic contents, and there is an increased echo behind the lesion. A few echos in the bottom of the tumor may emanate from a more solid part of the tumor. (From Pettersson et al. 1985b, with permission.)

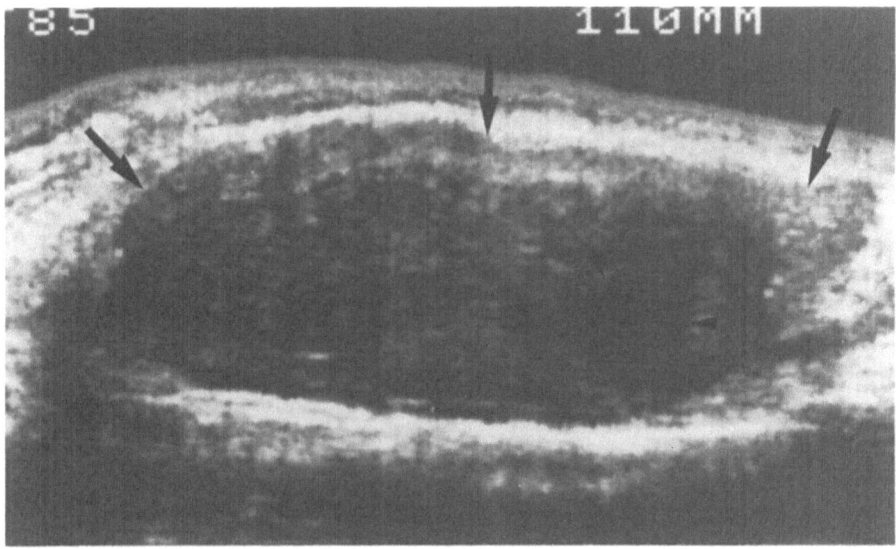

Fig. 6.12. Solid lesion: ultrasound. Female, 20 years, neurofibroma of the thigh. In the posterior thigh there is a large lesion (*arrows*) with mixed echogenicity, consistent with a solid tumor. In the distal part of the tumor there is a non-echogenic area consistent with cyst formation (*arrowheads*).

are detected by their very strong echos and the presence of a "shadow" behind them. But again, ultrasound has generally been used only seldom in the diagnostic work-up of musculoskeletal tumors (Bernardino et al. 1981).

Angiography

The diagnostic capabilities of angiography are limited, for both bone and soft tissue tumors. Even though the angiographic patterns of several bone and soft tissue tumors are characteristic, and a few, such as those of an angiolipoma or a cavernous venous hemangioma, are nearly pathognomonic (Fig. 4.1), the overlap between different tumor types is considerable (Levine et al. 1979). We have found the method of little value in the differential diagnosis of musculoskeletal sarcomas (Enneking 1983).

Scintigraphy

In the evaluation of the tumor matrix ^{99m}Tc-scintigraphy may reveal necrotic (cold) areas in a malignant tumor with otherwise increased uptake (Enneking et al. 1981) (Fig. 6.13). As an aid to the specific diagnosis the method is of limited value, but some patterns have been reported. Thus, in osteoid osteoma scintigraphy may be useful not only in detecting the lesion and for preoperative and intraoperative localization of the tumor (Ghelman et al. 1981; Ghelman and Vigorita 1983), but also for specific diagnosis (Swee et al. 1979; Smith and Gilday 1980; Omojola et al. 1981; Helms et al. 1984). Helms et al. (1984), for instance, reported on a "double

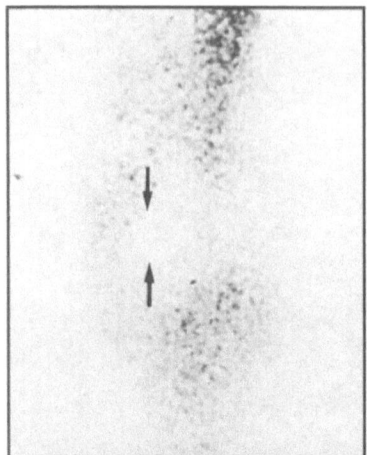

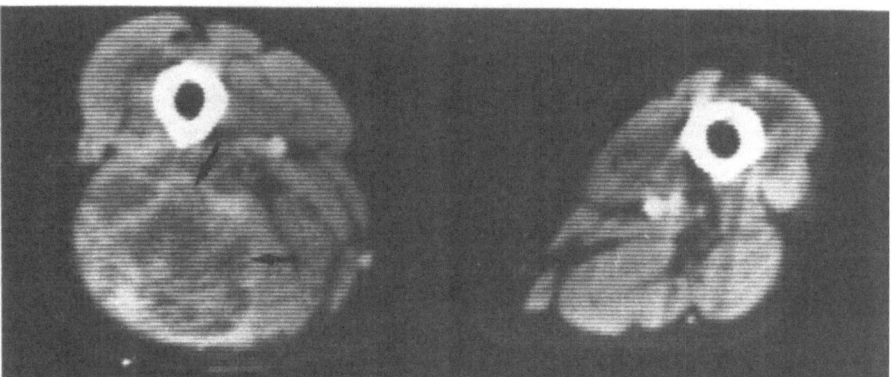

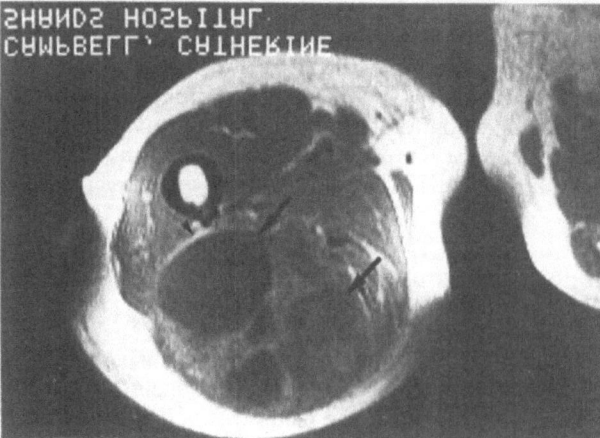

Fig. 6.13a–c. Soft tissue tumor with large central necrosis. **a** Scintigraphy, **b** CT, and **c** MRI. Female, 73 years, liposarcoma. **a** In the scintigraphic examination the necrosis is revealed as an area of decreased uptake (*arrows*). **b** In the CT image the necrosis is seen as areas of low attentuation (*arrows*). **c** In the T1-weighted MR image necrosis and liquefaction appear with low signal intensity (*arrows*). Note also the thin layer of fatty tissue between the tumor and the femur (*arrowhead*).

density sign": the nidus having a very high uptake, it was possible to delineate it in the area of increased uptake caused by the reactive rim. Other typical uptake patterns have also been reported. For example, a parosteal sarcoma and Ewing's sarcoma may have a more uniform uptake than a classical osteogenic sarcoma (Murray 1980), and giant cell tumors may have a rim of increased uptake around a photopenic area (Murray 1980; Peimer et al. 1980). But, generally, the information gained from scintigraphy is non-specific as to the diagnosis of the tumor.

Computed Tomography

Generally, CT is regarded as less suitable for the specific diagnosis of *bone tumors* than are plain films (Coenen et al. 1978; Levine et al. 1979; Rosenthal 1985), but there are several important exceptions to this rule. Calcifications are detected more sensitively than at plain film examination (Fig. 6.14), and also faint diffuse calcification or ossification may be revealed because of the high attenuation value of the

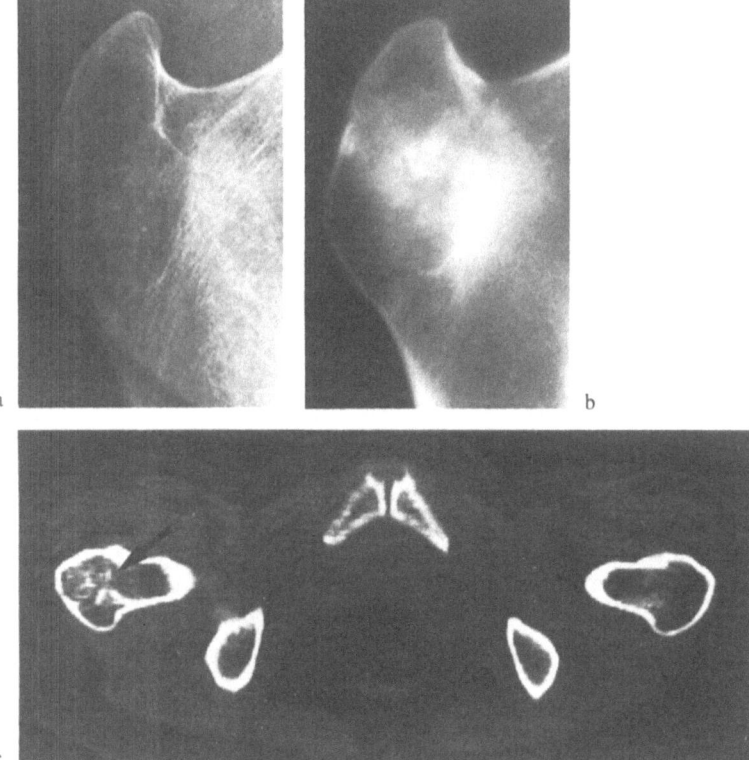

Fig. 6.14a–c. Intraosseous calcifications: comparison between plain film, conventional tomography, and CT. Male, 53 years, chondrosarcoma of the greater trochanter. **a** In the plain film examination the calcifications are barely visible. **b** With conventional tomography the area of calcification is more obvious. **c** CT clearly reveals the calcified lesion (*arrow*).

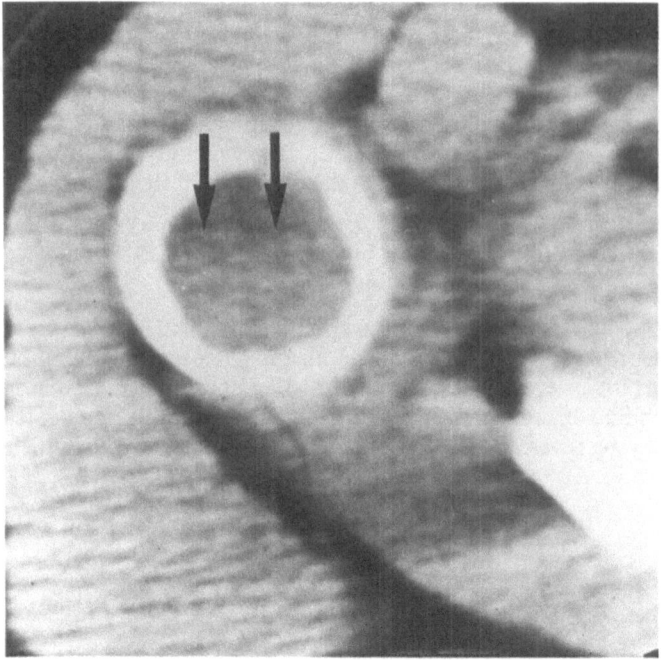

Fig. 6.15. Fluid–fluid level: CT. Female, 20 years, aneurysmal bone cyst. The fluid–fluid level (*arrows*) is not seen until after 20–30 min of rest.

lesion—usually values above 100 Hounsfield units (HU) mean a calcifying or ossifying tumor (Hudson 1986). Aneurysmal bone cysts contain variable proportions of solid and liquid components and appear inhomogeneous on the CT image. However, fluid–fluid levels forming within the tumor during rest have been described as an almost pathognomonic sign both in this tumor and in the much less common telangiectatic osteosarcoma (Hudson 1984) (Fig. 6.15).

Areas of necrosis and liquefaction have a low density, with attentuation values around zero, and in most cases are easy to differentiate from the tumor. But technical factors may make the evaluation of cystic contents hazardous: only in properly calibrated scanners is the attenuation of water zero and small errors in the attenuation values may be misleading. Rosenthal (1985) has therefore suggested that the attenuation of suspected cysts should be compared with the values of the surrounding muscle. Cysts should then have a value approximately 30–40 HU less than that of the muscle.

Outside the central nervous system the presence or absence of enhancement after intravenous injection or infusion of contrast medium is dependent on the vascularity of the tissue and is therefore of diagnostic value. Poorly vascularized tumors, such as those composed of cartilage, will not show enhancement, nor will areas of necrosis or liquefaction. Richly vascularized tumors, however, such as giant cell tumor, round cell tumor and Ewing's sarcoma, show considerable enhancement (Fig. 6.16); often an increase of 25–50 HU may be seen using the infusion technique described earlier (Hudson et al. 1984).

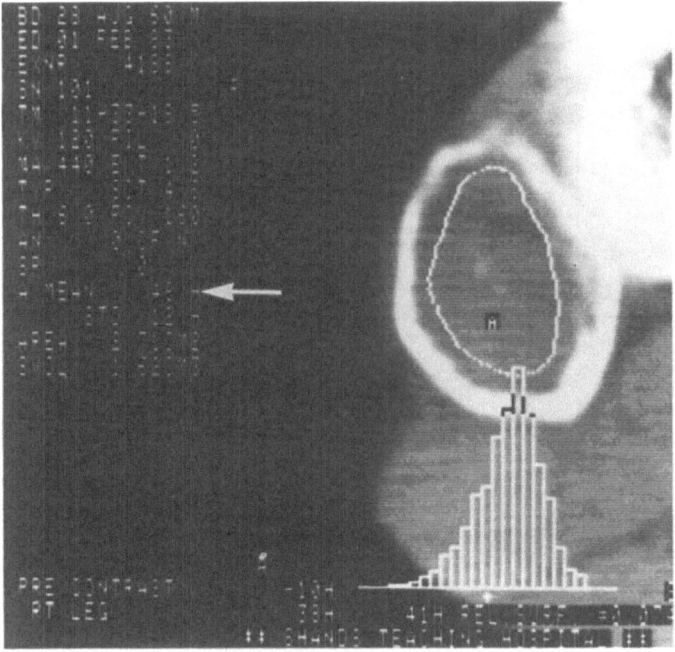

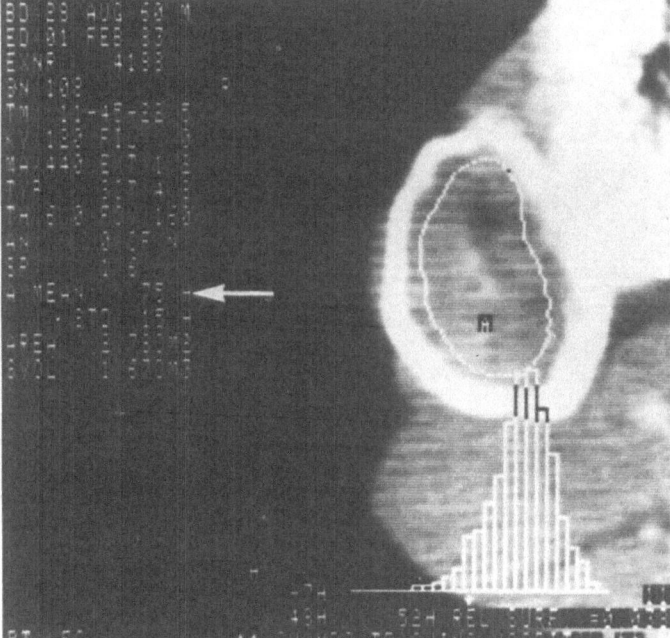

Fig. 6.16a,b. Tumor enhancement: CT. Male, 20 years, giant cell tumor of the fibular head. **a** Before contrast medium infusion. The mean attenuation value in the region of interest, marked with a cursor, is 48 HU (*arrow*). The histogram below the image of the fibula gives the distribution of the attenuation. **b** During contrast medium infusion. The attenuation value has increased to 75 HU (*arrow*).

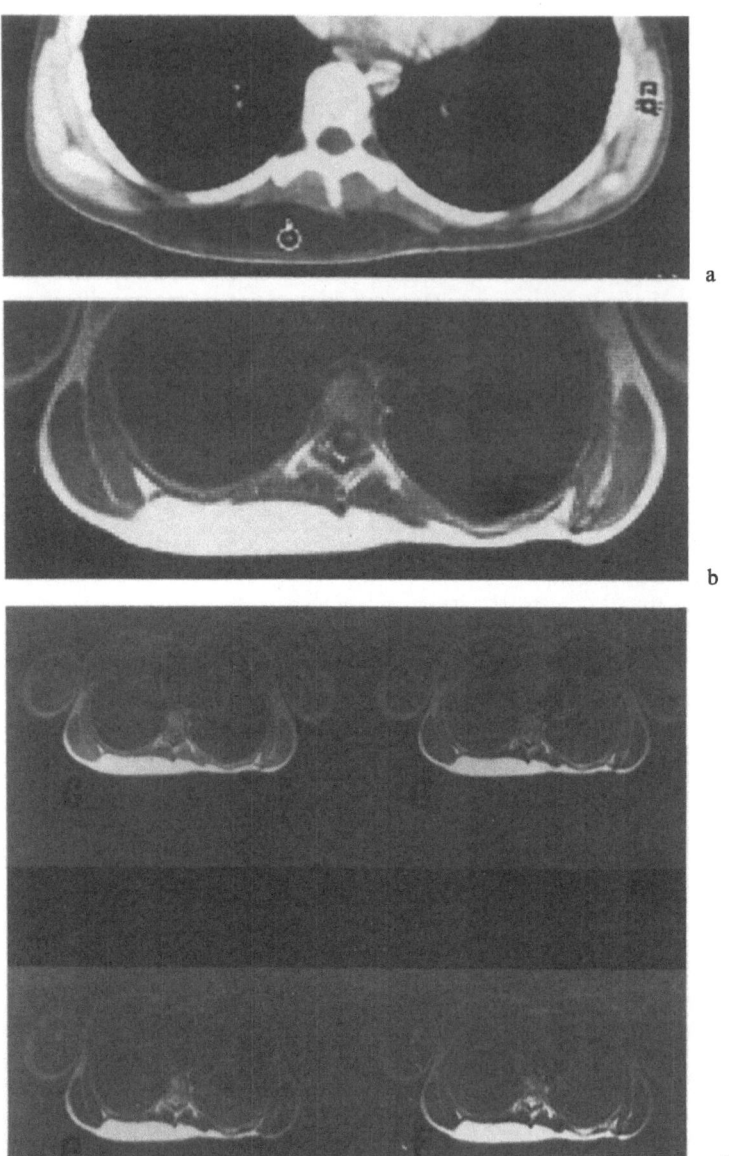

a

b

c–f

Fig. 6.17a–f. Lipoma: CT and MRI. Female, 17 years. **a** The CT examination reveals a lesion in the back with low attenuation (−75 HU) that is not enhanced during intravenous infusion of contrast medium. The findings are pathognomonic for a lipoma. **b** MRI, SE 500/30 ms (T1-weighted); and **c–f** MRI, SE 500/30, /60, /90, /120 ms (T2-weighted).

In all sequences the signal intensity from the lesion is equal to that from the subcutaneous fat. This is also pathognomonic for a lipoma. (From Pettersson et al. 1985a, with permission.)

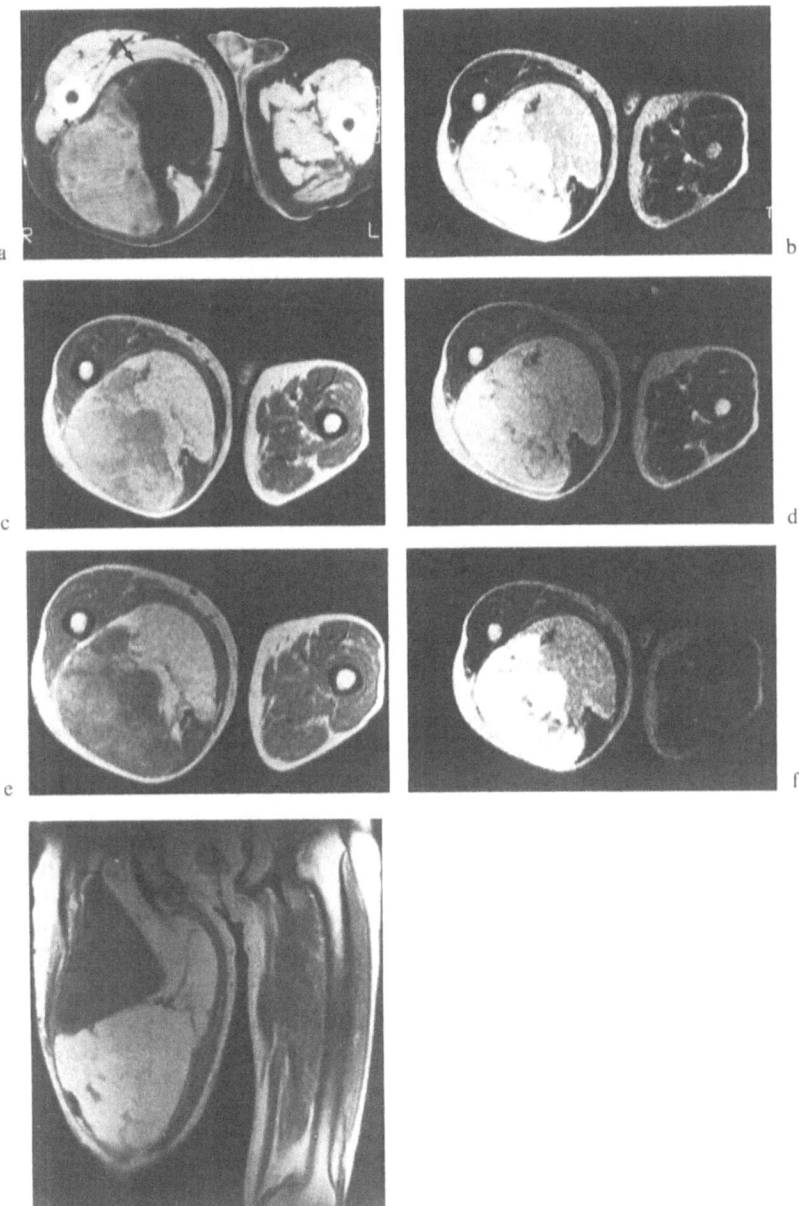

Fig. 6.18a–g. Liposarcoma: CT and MRI. Same patient as Fig. 5.18. **a** The CT image clearly differs between the low-density portion of the tumor that contains only benign lipomatous tissue (*arrows*) and the sarcomatous, enhanced malignant portion (*arrowheads*). **b** MRI, SE 500/30 ms, transaxial section (T1-weighted). **c–f** MRI, SE 2000/30, /60, /90, /120 ms (T2-weighted). **g** MRI, SE 500/30 ms, coronal section (T1-weighted).

In the T1-weighted images the sarcomatous portion has about the same signal intensity as the surrounding muscle, while in the T2-weighted sequence the signal intensity increases with increasing TE (30⟶120 ms). In all sequences the lipomatous portion of the tumor has the same signal intensity as the subcutaneous fat.

In *soft tissue tumors*, CT has a considerable potential for tissue characterization, due to the high contrast resolution of soft tissue that it affords. It has proved to be diagnostic for lipoma due to the low attenuation of this tumor. Thus, a homogeneous well-demarcated tumor with attenuation values varying between -60 HU and -100 HU that is not enhanced during intravenous infusion of contrast medium can safely be diagnosed as a benign lipoma, even if it contains thin strands of denser tissue (Fig. 6.17) (Hunter et al. 1979). Liposarcomas contain discrete areas of increased density (Hunter et al. 1979; Ekelund et al. 1982) (Fig. 6.18). If the lesion has ill-defined margins bordering the surrounding tissue, an infiltrative lipoma (Dionne and Seeymayer 1974) is probable (Rosenthal 1982). CT may also be diagnostic for pseudomalignant osseous tumor of soft parts, also known as myositis ossificans. The calcified periphery of this lesion, a center of low density, and the absence of any soft tissue component outside the calcification, are all changes that can easily be defined at the CT examination. As for bone tumors, the method can be used to define cystic lesions and areas of necrosis (Figs. 6.13b and 6.19a). Tumors of vascular origin may be enhanced considerably, and even vessels within the tumor may be visualized.

Magnetic Resonance Imaging

The contrast discrimination of soft tissue provided by MRI far exceeds that of any other imaging modality. This has proved to be great of importance for the assessment of the local extension of musculoskeletal tumors, as will be discussed in Chapter 7. However, as regards diagnosis, this aspect of MRI has so far added only little to the possibilities provided by CT. A lipoma may be diagnosed as having the same signal intensity as the surrounding normal fat in all pulse sequences (Fig. 6.17b–f) (Pettersson et al. 1985a), and the malignant areas can easily be identified in a liposarcoma that contains both fatty and sarcomatous tissue (Fig. 6.18). Areas of necrosis, hemorrhage and liquefaction can also be defined, even better than by CT (Figs. 6.13c and 6.19b,c). Fluid–fluid level in aneurysmal bone cysts are seen as accurately as with CT (Fig. 6.20). Calcifications have no magnetic resonance signal and appear black on the image; however, they are not as well visualized by MRI as by CT (Zimmer et al. 1985) (Fig. 6.21).

Tissue Characterization: T1 and T2 Values

For diagnostic purposes, MRI affords a potential that is very interesting and indeed opens up a new dimension in diagnostic imaging: tissue characterization based on T1 and T2 relaxation values.

Since the initial observation by Damadian (1971) of elevated T1 values in sarcomas, there have been a vast number of reports based on spectroscopic measurements of the substantial change in T1 and T2 relaxation characteristics in malignant tissue. MRI of musculoskeletal tumors is still in its infancy, and little is known about the tissue characterization of these lesions in vivo.

This tissue characterization can be approached in two ways. As the signal intensity seen on the image is determined mainly by proton density and relaxation times, one way is just to look at the magnetic resonance picture in the way one would evaluate a traditional radiologic image. In this way lipomas, necrosis, hemorrhage

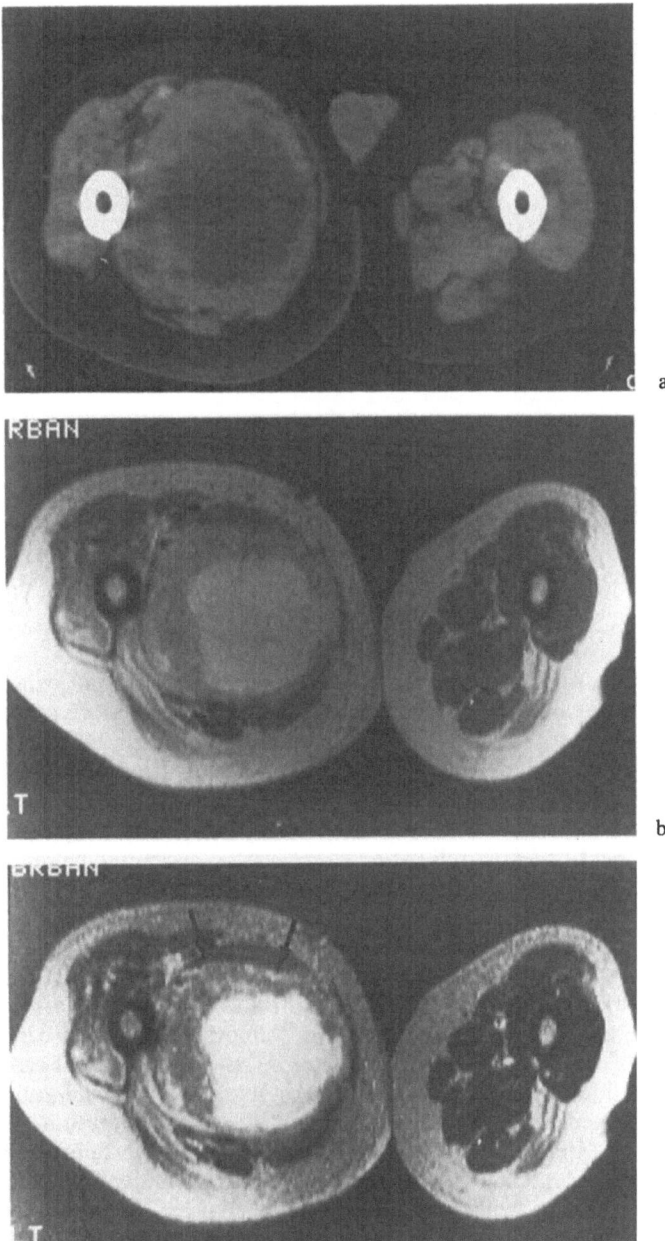

Fig. 6.19a–c. Necrosis and liquefaction: CT and MRI. Male, 70 years, malignant fibrous histiocytoma of the thigh. **a** The CT examination reveals the large tumor with a big central low-density area, consistent with necrosis and liquefaction. Because of edema and pressure effect on the muscle, the border between tumor and normal muscle cannot be defined. **b** MR image, SE 2500/45 ms, and **c** MR image, SE 2500/180 ms. In these two T2-weighted images the signal from the necrotic area is intense. It is also easy to delineate the vital tumor from the surrounding, normal muscle (*arrows*). (From Pettersson et al. 1985a, with permission.)

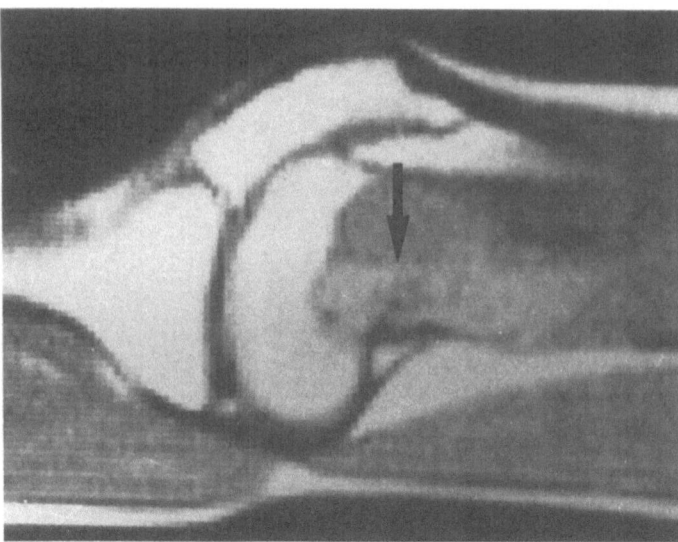

Fig. 6.20. Fluid–fluid level: MRI. Male, 18 years, aneurysmal bone cyst in the distal femur. The level is clearly seen (*arrow*).

and liquefaction may be identified as described above, but in most cases the visual approach is not adequate for making any differential diagnosis. The more exact way of studying the tissue characterization is to calculate the T1 and T2 values from the magnetic resonance image. This method has now been tried in clinical practice (Pettersson et al. 1985d; Zimmer et al. 1985).

In an attempt to assess the value of T1 and T2 measurements for diagnostic purposes, we calculated the T1 and T2 relaxation times in 58 consecutive patients with histologically verified musculoskeletal tumors (Pettersson et al. 1985d). The values found were correlated with the histopathologic diagnosis. All tumors except lipomas had relaxation values far above those of muscle, fat and bone marrow. The values for lipoma did not differ from that for normal fat. There was a statistically significant difference in mean values for both the T1 and T2 relaxation times between some of the different groups of musculoskeletal tumors. However, in each tumor group the range of values was wide and, therefore, in the individual case the relaxation values could not be used for differential diagnosis. One explanation for this could be the heterogeneity of the tumor matrix of musculoskeletal tumors. We found no direct correlation between the histologic grade and the relaxation value. However, these findings are only to be regarded as early results, and with further research this new modality will probably contribute a large amount of new information to the diagnostic work-up, especially when combined with spectroscopy.

Nuclear Magnetic Resonance Spectroscopy

The most accurate way to analyze tissue using nuclear magnetic resonance is spectroscopy. A malignancy index based on both T1 and T2 relaxation times has proved

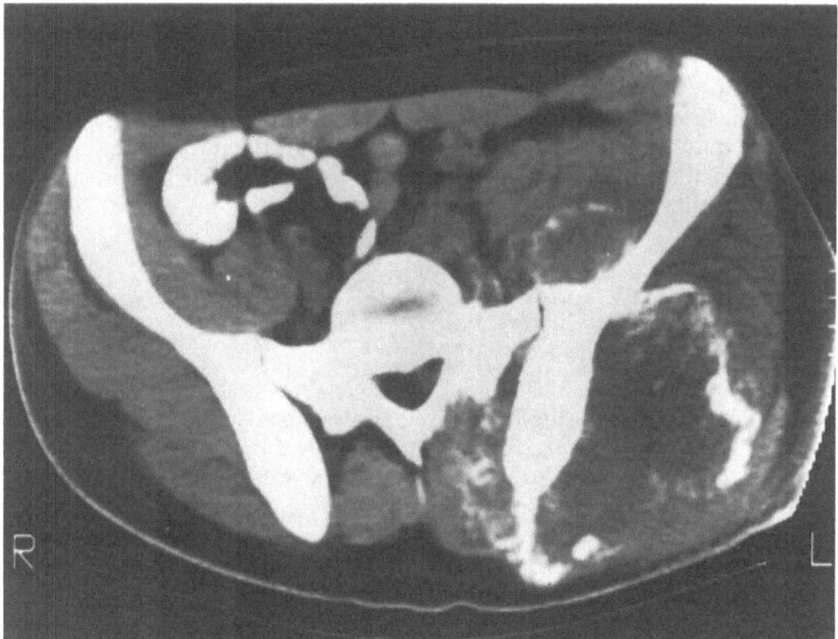

a

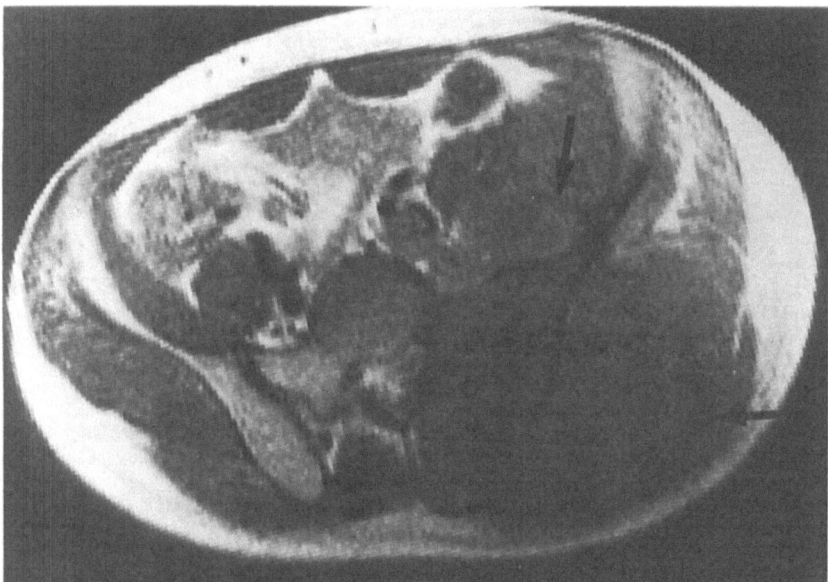

b

Fig. 6.21a,b. Soft tissue calcifications: CT and MRI. Male, 17 years, osteogenic sarcoma during chemotherapy. Same patient as Fig. 4.7. **a** The CT examination reveals extensive calcification/ ossification. **b** MRI, SE 500/30 ms (T1-weighted). Calcifications have almost no signal intensity and therefore appear black. The pronounced calcification can barely be identified in the MR image (*arrows*).

to be very accurate in differentiating between benign and malignant tissue in vitro, for both bone and soft tissue specimens (Koutcher et al. 1978). In such spectroscopy, phosphorus-31 has become important because of the element's metabolic significance: its use allows both the composition and metabolism of the tumor to be analyzed. The first reports on such studies in vivo (Griffiths et al. 1983; Nidecker et al. 1985) are quite encouraging, and it is possible that the information on both composition and metabolism of the tumor derived from such studies may be important for diagnosis and follow-up of tumor patients.

The Diagnosis

A meticulous analysis of the criteria discussed above and a synthesis of all the findings provide the basis for diagnosis. Bone tumors, being more available for analysis at plain film radiography than soft tissue tumors, have been thoroughly studied for generations and their characteristics as to the different criteria are well known. An example of the characteristics of the more common bone tumors, as found in plain film radiography, is given in Table 6.1 (Kricun 1983). As mentioned already, the diagnosis may be more difficult for soft tissue tumors.

References

Bernardino ME, Jing BS, Thomas JL, Lindell MM, Zornoza J (1981) The extremity soft-tissue lesion: A comparative study of ultrasound, computed tomography and xeroradiography. Radiology 139: 53–59

Blair RJ, McAfee JG (1976) Radiological detection of skeletal metastases: Radiographs versus scans. Int J Radiat Oncol Biol Phys 1: 1201–1205

Citrin DL, Bessent RG, Greig WR (1977) A comparison of the sensitivity and accuracy of the ^{99m}Tc-phosphate bone scan and skeletal radiograph in the diagnosis of bone metastases. Clin Radiol 28: 107–117

Coenen Y, Marchal G, Baert AL, Wilms G, Termote JL, Van Dooren W, Ponette E (1978) Contribution of computer tomography in the evaluation of bone tumors and associated pathology. J Belg Radiol 61: 399–403

Dahlin DC (1978) Bone tumors. Charles C Thomas, Springfield, Illinois

Damadian RV (1971) Tumor detection by nuclear magnetic resonance. Science 171: 1151–1153

Dionne GP, Seeymayer TA (1974) Infiltrating lipomas and angiolipomas revisited. Cancer 33: 732

Edeiken J (1983) Roentgen diagnosis of diseases of bone, 3rd edn. Williams and Wilkins, Baltimore

Ekelund L, Herrlin K, Rydholm A (1982) Comparison of computed tomography and angiography in the evaluation of soft tissue tumors of the extremities. Acta Radiol [Diagn] 23: 15–28

Enneking WF (1977) Clinical musculoskeletal pathology. Storter Printing Company, Gainesville, Florida, pp 315–320

Enneking WF (1983) Musculoskeletal tumor surgery. Churchill Livingstone, Edinburgh, pp 69–168

Enneking WF, Kagan A (1975) "Skip" metastases in osteosarcoma. Cancer 36: 2191–2193

Enneking WF, Chew FS, Springfield DS, Hudson TM, Spanier SS (1981) The role of radionuclide bone-scanning in determining the resectability of soft-tissue sarcomas. J Bone Joint Surg [Am] 63: 249–257

Feldman F, Hecht HC, Johnston AD (1970) Chondromyxoid fibroma of bone. Radiology 94: 249–260

Ghelman B, Vigorita VJ (1983) Postoperative radionuclide evaluation of osteoid osteomas. Radiology 146: 508–512

Ghelman B, Thompson FM, Arnold WD (1981) Intraoperative radioactive localization of an osteoid osteoma. J Bone Joint Surg [Am] 63: 826–827

Gilday DL, Ash JM, Reilly BJ (1977) Radionuclide skeletal survey for pediatric neoplasms. Radiology 123: 399–406

Goldstein H, McNeil BJ, Zufall E, Jaffe MB, Treves S (1980) Changing indications for bone scintigraphy in patients with osteosarcoma. Radiology 135: 177–180

Griffiths JR, Cady E, Edwards RHT et al. (1983) ^{31}P-NMR studies of a tumor in situ. Lancet I: 1435–1436

Helms CA, Hattner RS, Vogler JB III (1984) Osteoid osteoma: Radionuclide diagnosis. Radiology 151: 779–784

Hudson TM, Schiebler M, Springfield DS, Enneking WF, Hawkins IF Jr., Spanier SS (1984) Radiology of giant cell tumors of bone: Computed tomography, arthrotomography and scintigraphy. Skeletal Radiol 11: 85–95

Hudson TM (1984) Fluid levels in aneurysmal bone cysts: A CT feature. AJR 141: 1001–1004

Hudson TM (1986) Radiologic-pathologic correlation of musculoskeletal lesions. Williams and Wilkins, Baltimore (in press)

Hunter JC, Johnston WH, Genant HK (1979) Computed tomography evaluation of fatty tumors of the somatic soft tissues: Clinical utility and radiologic-pathologic correlation. Skeletal Radiol 4: 79–91

Johnson LC (1953) A general theory of bone tumors. Bull NY Acad Med 29: 164–172

Kirchner PT, Simon MA (1984) Current concepts review. Radioisotopic evaluation of skeletal disease. J Bone Joint Surg [Am] 63: 673–681

Koutcher JA, Goldsmith M, Damadian R (1978) NMR in cancer. X. A malignancy index to discriminate normal and cancerous tissue. Cancer 41: 174–182

Kricun ME (1983) Radiographic evaluation of solitary bone lesions. Arthritis Clin North Am 14: 39–64

Levine E, Lee KR, Neff JR, Maklad MF, Robinson RG, Preston DF (1979) Comparison of computed tomography and other imaging modalities in the evaluation of musculoskeletal tumors. Radiology 131: 431–437

Lodwick GS (1971) Atlas of tumor radiology. The bone and joints. Year Book Medical Publishers, Chicago, pp 65–79

Mangini U (1967) Tumors of the skeleton of the hand. Bull Hosp Joint Dis 28: 61–103

Martel W, Abell MR (1973) Radiologic evaluation of soft tissue tumors. Cancer 32: 352–366

McKillop JH, Etcubanas E, Goris ML (1981) The indications for and limitations of bone scintigraphy in osteogenic sarcoma. Cancer 48: 1133–1138

McLeod RA, Beabout JW (1973) The roentgenographic features of chondroblastoma. AJR 118: 464–471

McNeil BJ (1978) Rationale for the use of bone scans in selected metastatic and primary bone tumors. Semin Nucl Med 8: 336–345

Murray IP (1980) Bone scanning in the child and young adult. Skeletal Radiol 5: 1–14

Nidecker AC, Muller S, Aue WP et al. (1985) Extremity bone tumors: Evaluation by P-31 MR spectroscopy. Radiology 157: 167–174

Omojola MF, Cockshott WP, Beatty EG (1981) Osteoid osteoma: An evaluation of diagnostic modalities. Clin Radiol 32: 199–204

Peimer CA, Schiller AL, Mankin HJ (1980) Multicentric giant-cell tumor of bone. J Bone Joint Surg [Am] 62: 642–656

Pettersson H, Hamlin DJ, Mancuso A, Scott KN (1985a) Magnetic resonance imaging of the musculoskeletal system. Acta Radiol [Diagn] 26: 225–235

Pettersson H, Hudson TM, Springfield DS, Kaude JV (1985b) Cystic intramuscular myxoma. Acta Radiol [Diagn] 26: 425–426

Pettersson H, Hamlin DJ, Enneking WF, Springfield DS, Andrew ER, Spanier S, Slone R (1985c) MR imaging of primary musculoskeletal tumors: Experience from 193 examinations. Radiology 157(P): 109

Pettersson H, Spanier S, Fitzsimmons JR, Slone R, Scott KN (1985d) MR imaging relaxation measurements in musculoskeletal tumors and surrounding tissue. Radiology 157(P): 109

Rosenthal DI (1982) Computed tomography in bone and soft tissue neoplasms: Application and patho-
    logic correlation. CRC Crit Rev Diagn Imaging 18: 243–278
Rosenthal DI (1985) Computed tomography of orthopaedic neoplasms. Orthop Clin North Am 16:
    461–470
Smith FW, Gilday DL (1980) Scintigraphic appearances of osteoid osteoma. Radiology 137: 191–195
Springfield DS, Enneking WF, Neff JR, Mahley JT (1984) Principles of tumor management. In: Murray
    JA (ed) AAOS instructional course lectures. CV Mosby, St. Louis, pp 1–24
Swee RG, McLeod RA, Beabout JW (1979) Osteoid osteoma: Detection, diagnosis, and localization.
    Radiology 130: 117–123
Sweet DE, Madewell JE, Ragsdale BD (1981) Radiologic and pathologic analysis of solitary bone
    lesions. III. Matrix patterns. Radiol Clin North Am 19: 784–814
Wilner D (1982) Radiology of bone tumors and allied disorders. WB Saunders, Philadelphia, pp 25–75
Zimmer WD, Berquist TH, McLeod RA et al. (1985) Bone tumors: Magnetic resonance imaging versus
    computed tomography. Radiology 155: 709–718
Zlatkin MB, Lander PH, Begin LR, Hadjipavlou A (1985) Soft-tissue chondromas. AJR 144: 1263–1267

Chapter 7

Local Extent of the Tumor

Accurate determination of the exact anatomic extent of the tumor and its reaction is a prerequisite of rational surgical planning for all active and aggressive tumors. A meticulous radiologic examination of the extent of tumor should clarify the following parameters in great detail:

1. For bone tumors:
   a) intraosseous extent
   b) cortical breakthrough
   c) soft tissue component
   d) joint involvement
2. For soft tissue tumors and bone tumors with soft tissue extension:
   a) definition of involved compartment(s)
   b) involvement of the neurovascular bundle
   c) involvement of adjacent bone (for soft tissue tumors)

To achieve the answers to the above questions a combination of the diagnostic imaging modalities is often required. In this chapter the possibilities and limitations of the different modalities in this respect will be discussed.

Bone Tumors

Intraosseous Extent

On the *plain film examination* the longitudinal intraosseous extent of a latent lesion with a well-defined sclerotic rim is easy to detect (Fig. 5.6), and in such cases no more studies are necessary. In active and aggressive lesions the reactive zone is less well defined, and especially in aggressive lesions the exact border between the tumor and normal tissue may be impossible to identify (Fig. 5.8). The area of radiolucency may indicate the extent of tumor, and in cartilaginous tumors the area with pathologically calcified matrix may identify the extension (Fig. 7.1a) (Hudson et al. 1983a). However, using the plain film findings as a basis for evaluation of intraosseous extent entails a degree of uncertainty. The opinion as to how much bone of normal appearance proximal and distal to the lesion should be included in the resection or amputation varies between different tumor centers (Enneking and Springfield 1977).

Nowadays the plain film examination is vital for the evaluation of local behavior and for diagnosis, as discussed in earlier chapters, but as regards the evaluation of the intraosseous extent it should, in most cases, be used only in combination with other modalities.

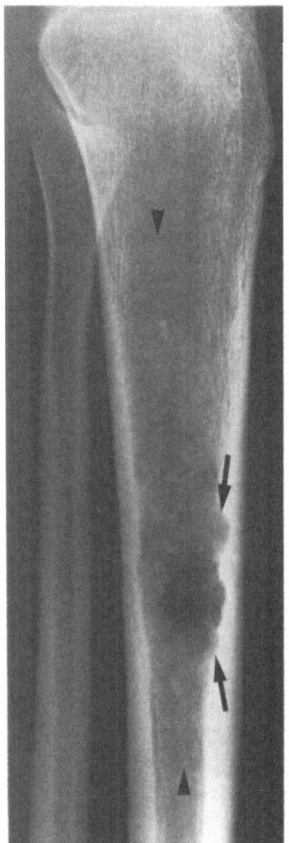
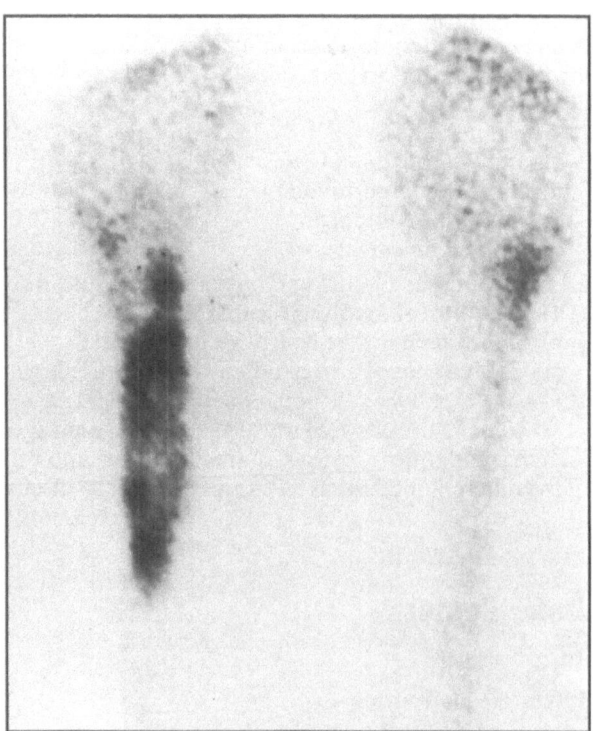

a   b

Fig. 7.1a–e. Intraosseous extent of tumor. Female, 50 years, chondrosarcoma. **a** Plain film radiograph. The tumor causes endosteal scalloping (*arrows*) and the longitudinal extent can be roughly estimated by the presence of the calcified tumor matrix (*arrowheads*). **b** Scintigraphy. The increased area of uptake may be used as a marker of tumor extent. **c** CT. The tumor has a much higher attenuation value than the bone marrow canal on the other side. However, the exact border between tumor and normal tissue may be impossible to identify with this method. **d** and **e** MRI, SE 500/30 ms, transaxial and sagittal sections. The tumor has a much lower signal intensity than the bone marrow, and is therefore easy to identify. Note the proximal extent of tumor in **e** (*arrow*), not possible to see with any of the other methods.

Conventional tomography has been used in the past to increase the information on the extent of the tumor. In recent reports it has also been found to be valuable, adding accurate information to plain film examinations of tumors (Hudson and Hawkins 1981; Hudson et al. 1983b).

Scintigraphy with bone-seeking substances may be used for the evaluation of tumor extent (Fig. 7.1b). However, not only the lesion itself but also the reactive zone around it may exhibit increased uptake, and differentiation between the lesion and the reactive zone is not possible by this method. Moreover, in aggressive lesions this area of increased uptake may extend well beyond both the tumor and the reactive zone—the "extended pattern of uptake" described by Thrall et al. (1975) or

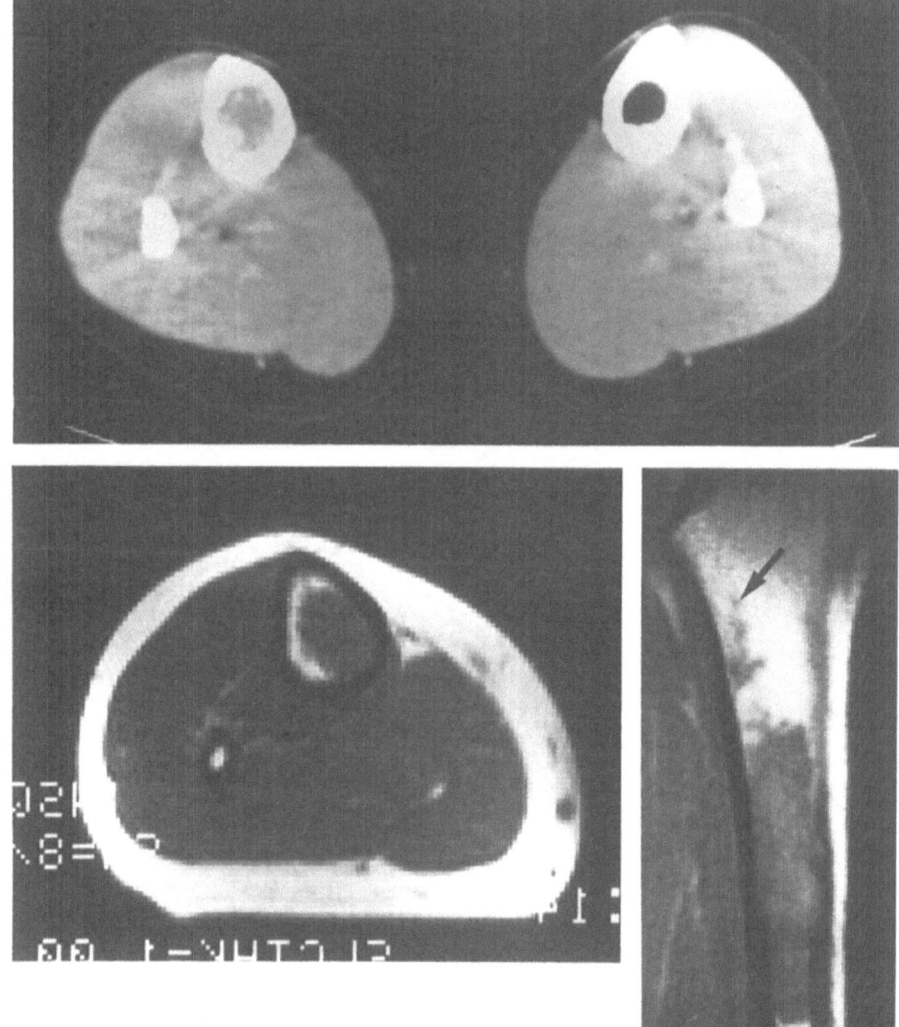

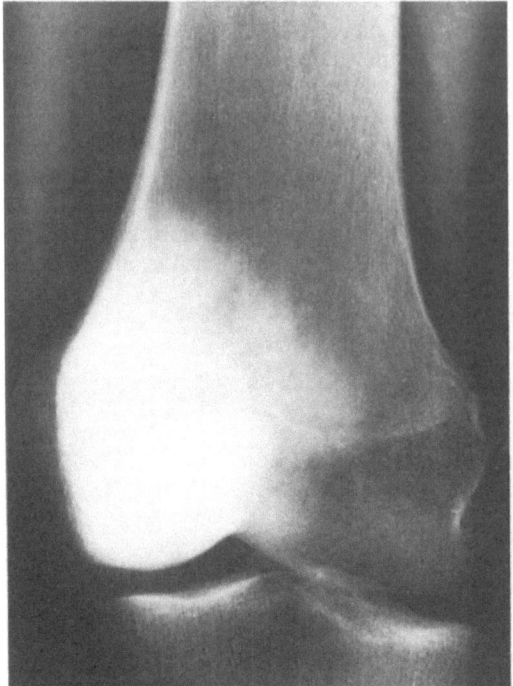

a

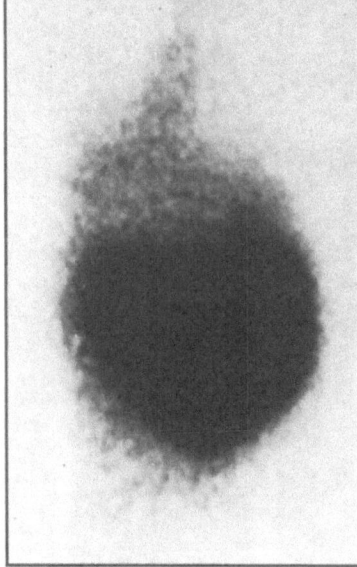

b

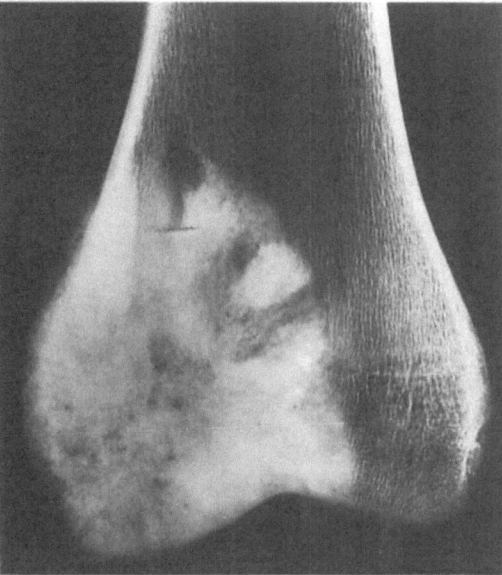

c

Fig. 7.2a–c. Extended pattern of uptake: scintigraphy. Male, 19 years, osteogenic sarcoma. **a** The preoperative plain film examination shows the dense, solid new bone formation, mainly in the medial condyle, with extension over the midline into the lateral condyle. **b** At scintigraphy there is intense uptake both in the medial and in most parts of the lateral condyle, in a larger area than would be anticipated from **a**. **c** The cut specimen reveals the true extent of tumor (as verified histologically). This extent is considerably smaller than that suggested by scintigraphy.

the "contiguous bone activity" of Simon and Kirchner (1980) (Fig. 7.2). Goldman and Braunstein (1975) and Thrall et al. (1975) have proposed that the reason for this extended zone could be the regional hyperemia, or osteopenia. Chew and Hudson (1982) in their study of osteosarcomas found the extended uptake to correspond to marrow hyperemia, medullary reactive bone and periosteal new bone formation. Extended uptake occurs much less frequently in medullary chondrosarcomas than in other aggressive bone tumors, possibly because chondrosarcomas are less vascular (Hudson et al. 1982).

In spite of the possible inconsistency between the scintigraphic extent and the true pathologic extent of tumor, this modality is used together with the plain film examination as an important tool in the evaluation of the intraosseous extent of tumor in the presurgical planning.

With *angiography* the intraosseous extent can be assessed accurately in highly vascularized tumors such as giant cell tumors, but others with pronounced vascularization, including osteosarcomas, may spread extensively along the medullary canal without producing any angiographic changes (Hudson and Hawkins 1981). In less vascularized tissue the spread is seen even less reliably. "Skip lesions" may be seen at angiography if their size is of the order of 1 cm or more, but by the time they have reached this size they are generally evident on the plain film (Enneking 1983).

With *computed tomography* the intramedullary extent of tumor can be clearly defined because of the higher attenuation values of tumor compared with the values of bone marrow in the normal contralateral limb (Figs. 4.6c and 7.1c). Using the digital radiograph as a map, the slices containing pathologic tissue can be defined, as can the distance between this tissue and the adjacent joints or any other landmarks (Fig. 4.6). Again, the reactive zone may cause difficulties, since it may also have increased attenuation values and may be enhanced after intravenous injection of contrast medium, just as the tumor. However, the problem of overestimating tumor extent seems to be less in CT examinations than in scintigraphy, and until the advent of MRI, CT and scintigraphy were the modalities of choice for the evaluation of tumor spread in the medullary canal (deSantos et al. 1979; Levine et al. 1979; Rosenthal 1985).

Reconstruction of the axial sections in the sagittal or coronal plane may display the extent more distinctly, but the spatial resolution in such imaging is poor and will add little to the information contained in the axial sections from which it derived (Fig. 4.6f).

CT has proved to be of great value in the evaluation of tumors within the pelvis, shoulder girdle and spine. Its value in these areas is increased because imaging in the axial plane gives important information on the relationship of the lesion to the paraspinal, intrapelvic and intrathoracic structures (Levine et al. 1979; Rosenthal 1982).

With *magnetic resonance imaging* the intraosseous extent is seen with a high degree of accuracy. The high contrast discrimination of soft tissue allows a more detailed definition of the tumor than does CT in the axial plane (Fig. 7.1d), and the possibility of imaging in any plane offers great advantage: imaging a few sections through the long bone parallel to its long axis gives exact information on the intraosseous extent (Figs. 7.1e and 7.3). The reactive zone has a different signal intensity from the tumor in both the T1- and T2-weighted images. In our experience MRI is the most accurate modality available for evaluation of the intraosseous extent of the tumor (Pettersson et al. 1985a; Reiser et al. 1984; Zimmer et al. 1985).

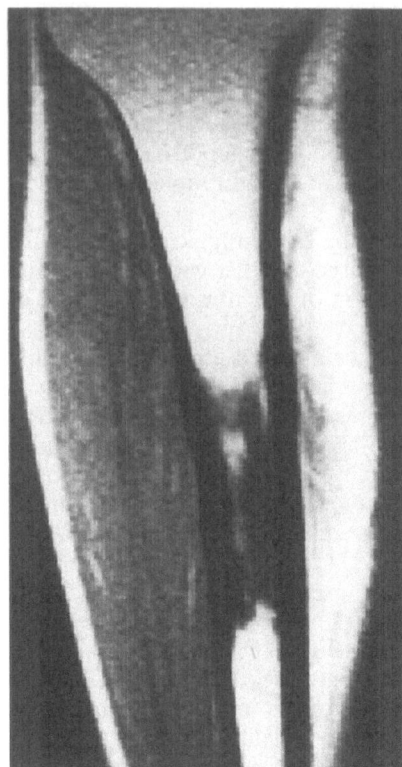

Fig. 7.3. Intraosseous tumor extent: MRI. Same patient as in Fig. 4.6. If the longitudinal plane is aligned exactly parallel with the long axis of the bone, it will reveal the longitudinal extent of the tumor in great detail.

Cortical Breakthrough

The mechanism of involvement of cortical bone by neoplastic tissue has been discussed in detail in connection with the local behavior of the tumor (Chapter 5). In the early stages of cortical destruction by intramedullary tumors only the inner part of the cortex may be involved, but as soon as the reactive zone reaches the outer surface there will be a corresponding periosteal reaction.

Plain film radiography in multiple projections is accurate for evaluation of the cortical bone. The examination reveals whether the cortex is thin, expanded, thickened, or fractured (Wilner 1982).

Small areas of cortical destruction are better seen by *computed tomography* using the bone window setting or bone algorithm, and most authors find CT superior to plain film radiography and conventional tomography in the evaluation of cortical integrity (Finkelstein 1975; deSantos et al. 1979; Hudson et al. 1984b).

With the instruments currently available, *magnetic resonance imaging* still has inferior spatial resolution compared with CT, and the cortical bone has no magnetic resonance signal. The contribution of MRI to the evaluation of cortical bone is therefore limited (Pettersson et al. 1985a; Zimmer et al. 1985). Highly aggressive malignant tumors with a permeative pattern of destruction (notably Ewing's sarcoma) may extend through the cortex without destroying the gross outline of the cortical bone, and in such cases MRI is of great value for detection of the soft tissue component, as will be discussed below.

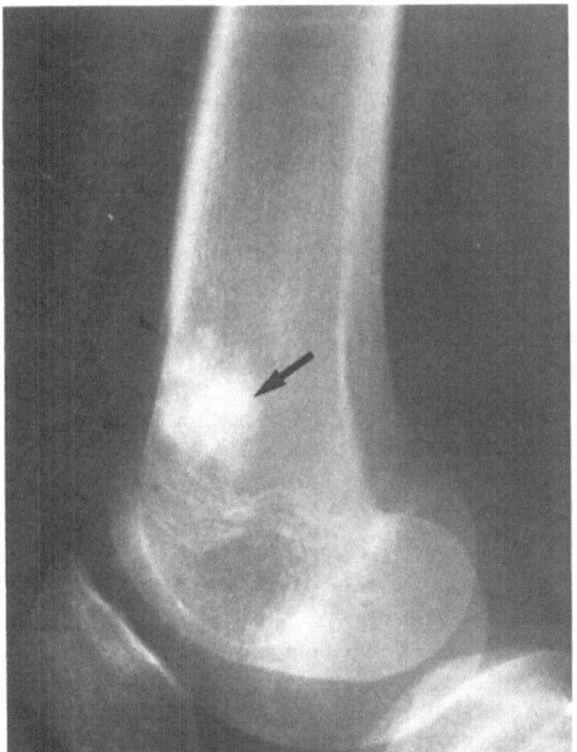

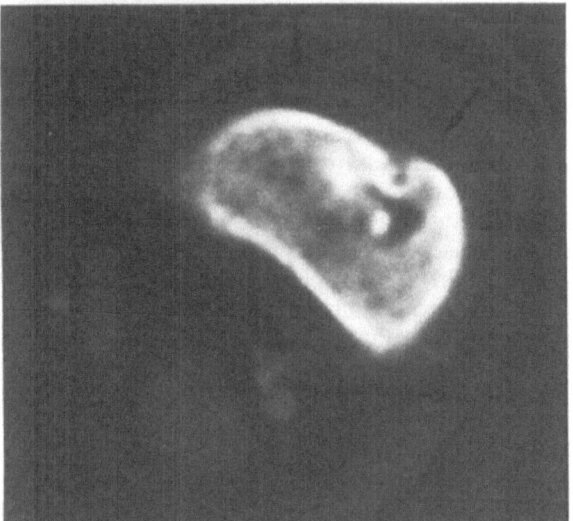

Fig. 7.4a,b. Edematous and inflammatory tissue, mimicking soft tissue extension of bone tumor at CT. Female, 20 years, osteogenic sarcoma. **a** Plain film examination. There is dense new bone formation in the distal femur (*arrow*) and possible cortical destruction (*arrowheads*), but no obvious soft tissue component of the tumor. **b** CT revals a soft tissue mass corresponding to the cortical breakthrough, interpreted as tumor (*arrows*). Pathologic examination revealed it to be only inflammatory tissue.

As regards the extraosseous part of bone tumours, plain films give an approximate estimate of the extension, especially when mineralization of the extraosseous matrix is seen (Figs. 5.16b and 6.7). Scintigraphy will give a more accurate estimate of the extent (Fig. 5.16a), and angiography may show the outline of the soft tissue extension. However, the best methods for evaluation of the extraosseous portion of bone tumors are CT and MRI. It is important to realize, though, that the soft tissue thickening around cortical bone as seen by CT can represent edematous reactive tissue and not true tumor (Fig. 7.4). MRI as well may be misleading in this respect, but with increased experience it may be possible to differentiate between inflammatory reaction and early extraosseous growth of bone tumor using MRI.

Soft Tissue Component

The radiology of the soft tissue component of bone tumors with extension outside the bone does not differ from that of soft tissue tumors. It will therefore be discussed below in connection with such tumors.

Joint Involvement

Tumor invasion of the adjacent joint is difficult to evaluate clinically, especially in its early stages. Simple aspiration to ascertain malignant diffusion is not reliable (DeSmet and Neff 1982), and capsular invasion cannot be excluded by the absence of effusion (Watts, 1980). *Plain film* examination may reveal destruction of the intra-articular cortical bone (Fig. 7.5a,b), but such destruction is better seen by *conventional tomography* (Fig. 7.5c) (Hudson et al. 1984b). However, even cortical breakthrough may not mean intra-articular involvement, as the cartilage and synovial lining may still be intact (Fig. 7.5d) (Hudson et al. 1984b).

DeSmet and Neff (1982), DeSmet et al. (1985) and Hudson et al. (1984b) have reported that *arthrography* combined with conventional tomography accurately reveals extension of bone tumor through both the cortex and the cartilage. This method is of value also for evaluation of intra-articular lesions such as synovial osteochondromatosis or pigmented villonodular synovitis. According to DeSmet et al. (1985) single contrast arthrography is best for detecting capsular impingement of soft tissue lesions, while double contrast arthrography is preferable for examining bone tumors that may penetrate into the joint or periosteal lesions that may be intra-articular. Because the tumor may potentially spread through the puncture canal, the injection site should be chosen so that in case of malignancy, it can be excised *en bloc* together with the tumor mass, as mentioned in Chapter 4. Arthrography should only be performed if the other methods do not give adequate information (DeSmet et al. 1985).

Computed tomography has been tried for evaluation of joint involvement (Soye et al. 1982) and has proved to be useful in selective cases. However, some joint surfaces, such as the inferior surface of the femoral condyles, the tibial condyles and the acetabular roof, are difficult or impossible to image in a plane perpendicular to the surface, and sections parallel to the joint surfaces are of limited value. In such cases conventional tomography is superior to CT.

The ease with which imaging in any plane can be performed with *magnetic resonance imaging* has been found to be of great value: sagittal or coronal sections

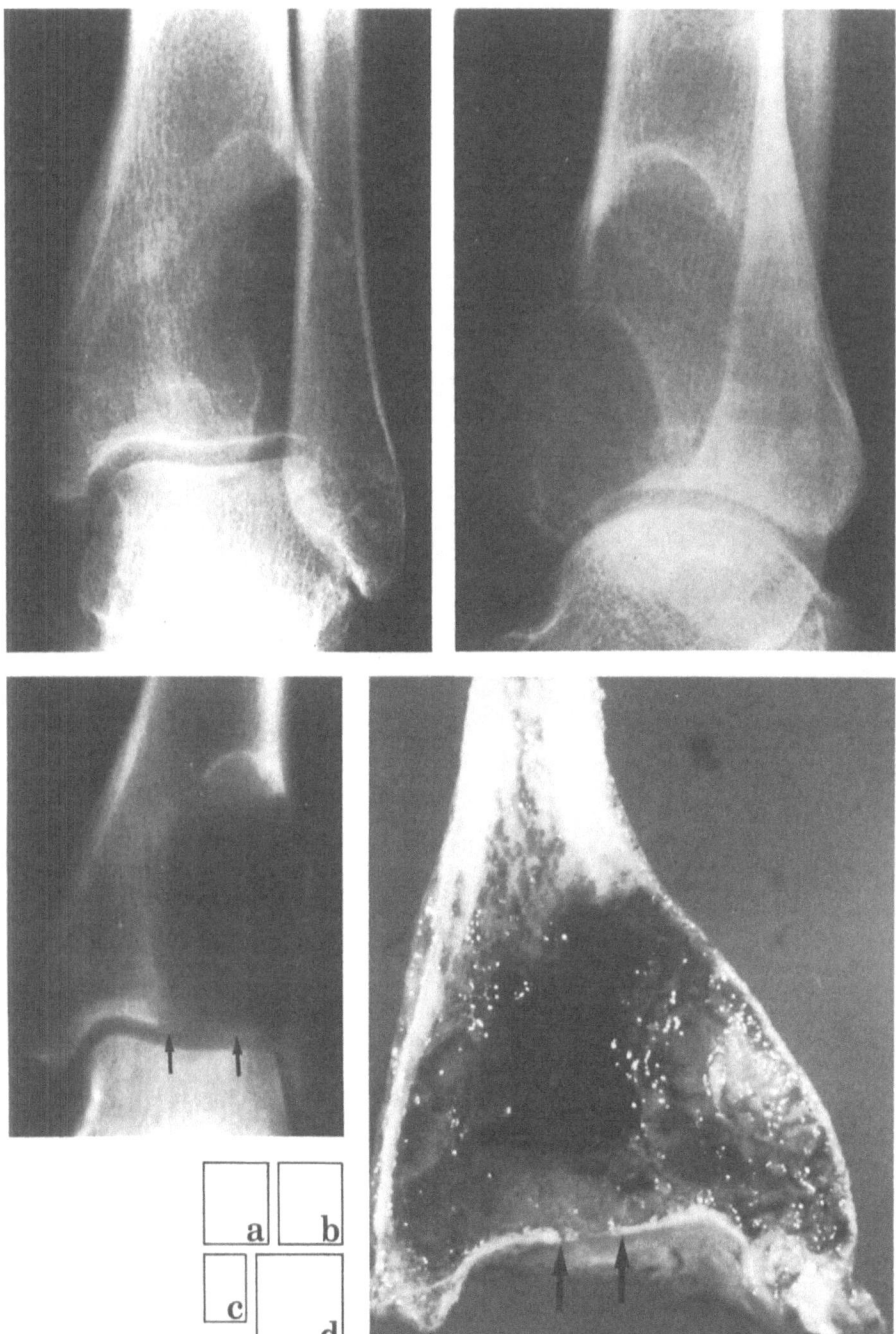

Fig. 7.5a–d. Evaluation of joint involvement: plain film and conventional tomography. Female, 15 years, giant cell tumor. **a** and **b** Plain film examination, AP and lateral. There is no definite breakthrough of the distal cortex. **c** Conventional tomography, AP, reveals destruction of the cortical bone (*between arrows*). **d** The specimen. The cartilage is preserved covering the cortical destruction (*between arrows*).

through, for instance, the knee reveal the outline of the cortex as well as the cartilage. In our experience this modality gives more information than any of the other non-invasive methods (Fig. 7.6) (Pettersson et al. 1985a), while others (Zimmer et al. 1985) have found MRI superior to CT only in a small percentage of cases. With increasing spatial resolution in the future, MRI will no doubt become the best method for evaluation of joint involvement.

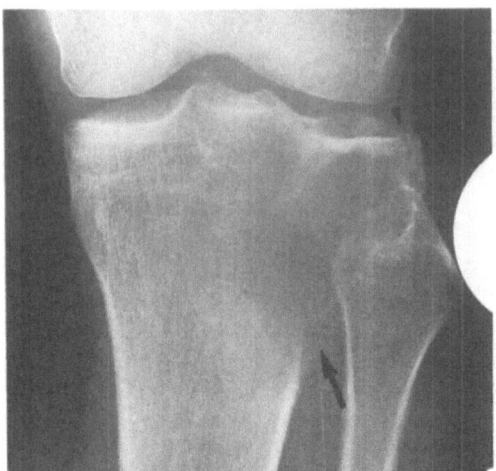

a

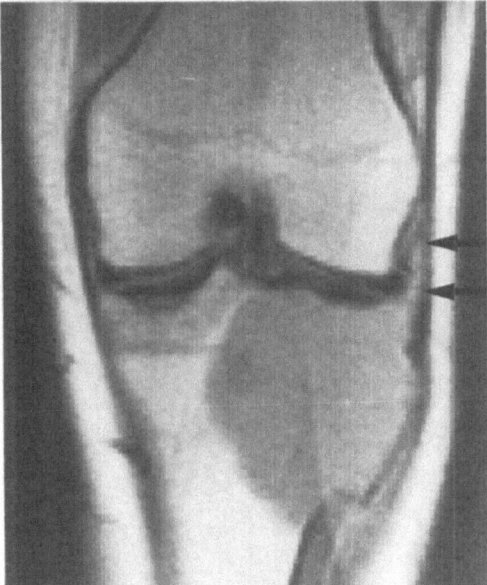

b

Fig. 7.6a,b. Joint involvement: plain film examination and MRI. Female, 26 years, giant cell tumor. **a** The plain film reveals the destruction of the lateral cortex (*arrows*) and the possible breakthrough at the most lateral part of the joint surface (*arrowhead*). **b** MRI, SE 500/30 ms, frontal section. The joint surface is intact, but there is extension of tumor along the collateral ligament (*arrows*).

Soft Tissue Tumors and Bone Tumors with Soft Tissue Extension

Definition of Involved Compartment(s)

For precise evaluation of the extent of soft tissue tumors, especially in the differentiation between different muscle compartments, plain films and scintigraphy are of limited value.

Prior to the advent of CT and MRI, *angiography* was used to determine whether the soft tissue component of a lesion was intra- or extracompartmental. However, although the experienced radiologist can make such a determination with high accuracy (Enneking 1983), the best methods today are CT and MRI.

In this respect, *computed tomography*, because of its high contrast resolution, has revolutionized the traditional methods (Rosenthal 1982, 1985). With contrast-enhanced high-resolution CT, muscle groups, bone and subcutaneous tissue can easily be differentiated. The major neurovascular bundles are clearly visible, although the nerve may be difficult to identify (Fig. 7.7). As many tumors have attenuation values that differ from those of normal muscle and fat, the outline of the lesion is often possible to define, and the fat-containing fascial planes between the muscle compartments help in the localization (Fig. 7.8). Several tumors, however, may have attenuation values very near that of muscle, both before and after contrast enhancement. In such instances the tumor will be visible only as an enlargement of the muscle, if it is detectable at all (Fig. 7.9a). Moreover, soft tissue planes between the different compartments may be obliterated by pressure and/or edema, making evaluation of the compartmentalization of the tumor difficult, even when

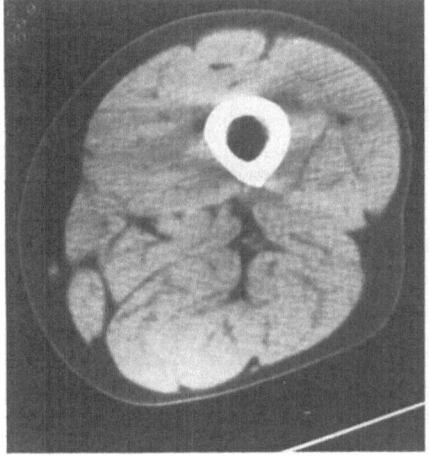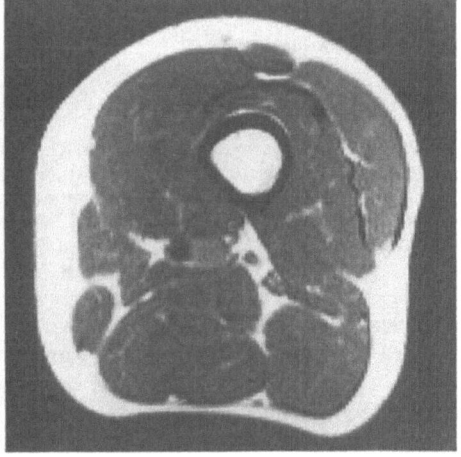

a   b

Fig. 7.7a,b. Normal thigh: **a** CT and **b** MRI taken on the same occasion. Male, 43 years. The muscle groups, subcutaneous fat, bone, large vessels and nerves are well delineated with both methods, but the soft tissue contrast discrimination is higher with MRI than CT.

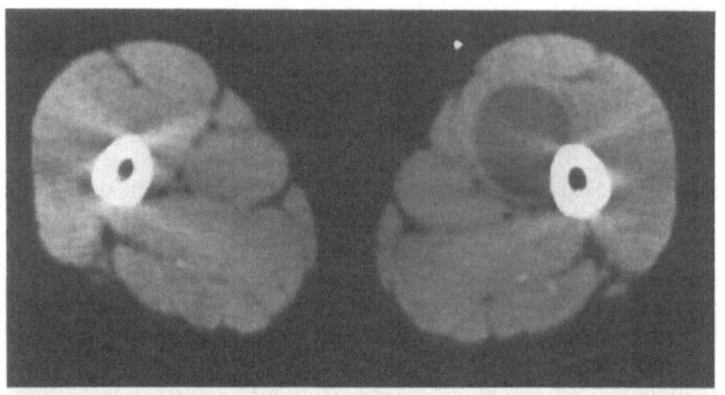

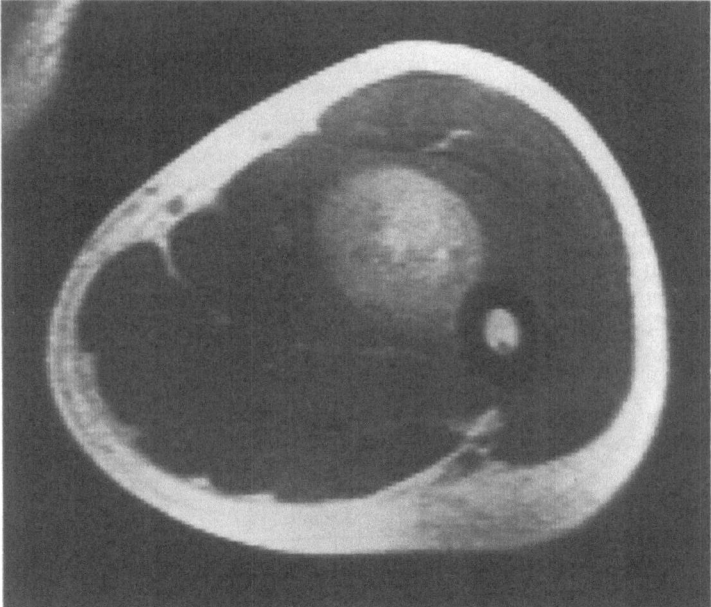

Fig. 7.8a,b. Soft tissue tumor: **a** CT and **b** MRI. Male, 18 years, neurofibroma. **a** In the CT examination the tumor has a considerably lower attenuation value than the surrounding muscle, and the fat in the fascial planes makes localization of the tumor easy. There is no tissue plane between the tumor and the bone. **b** MRI, SE 2000/30 ms. In this T2-weighted image the high signal intensity of the tumor differentiates it from surrounding muscle and bone. The information as to localization is the same as in **a**.

it is clearly visible. It has been shown that the edema and inflammatory reaction around the tumor can mimic the tumor itself at CT, thus making differentiation between the malignant tissue and the surrounding normal muscle or fat difficult (Fig. 6.19a) (Egund et al. 1981; Jones and Kuhns 1981; Ekelund et al. 1982; Golding and Husband 1982).

Magnetic resonance imaging has provided a considerable improvement over CT. Normal soft tissue structures are even better visualized than with CT. Using SE sequences the signal intensity of soft tissue tumors in the T1-weighted images often

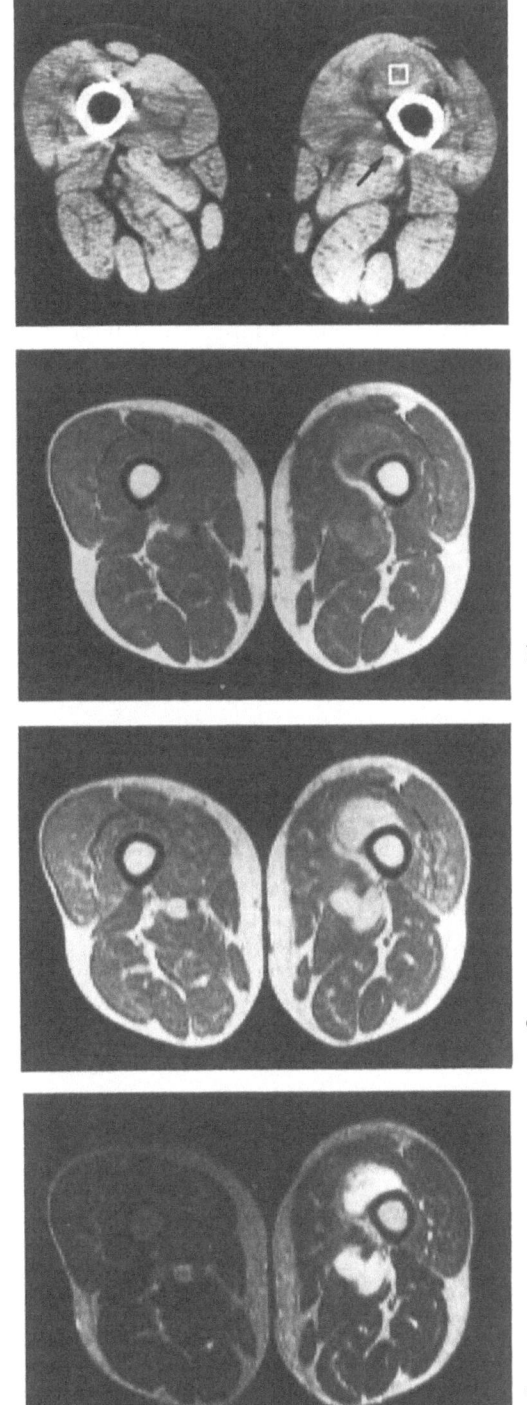

Fig. 7.9a–d. Soft tissue tumor: **a** CT and **b–d** MRI. Male, 47 years, mixed liposarcoma. **a** In the CT examination the tumor is detectable as an increase in the size of vastus musculature, with slightly decreased attenuation. It is not possible to assess the relation between tumor and bone or tumor and vessel (*arrow*). **b–d** MRI, SE 500/30 (**b**), 2000/30 (**c**) and 2000/90 ms (**d**). While the T1-weighted image (**b**) depicts the normal anatomy, the T2-weighted images (**c,d**) clearly define the tumor. The lesion is immediately adjacent to the bone and the neurovascular bundle is involved. (From Pettersson et al. 1985b, with permission.)

equals that of muscle. These sequences provide good discrimination between tumor and fat, while the delineation between muscle and tumor is poor (Figs. 4.8a and 7.9b). In the T2-weighted images the signal intensity of the tumor is high, and differs very clearly from the signal of the muscle (Figs. 4.8b–e and 7.9c,d) (Brady et al. 1983; Moon et al. 1983; Hudson et al. 1985; Pettersson et al. 1985a,b; Reiser et al. 1984; Zimmer et al. 1985). Necrosis and liquefaction also have signals that differ from that of tumor. Therefore, with MRI there is considerably less difficulty than with CT in differentiating tumor, necrosis and normal muscle (Fig. 6.19b,c) (Pettersson et al. 1985a,b).

MRI has another significant advantage over CT in the evaluation of tumor extent: easy imaging in the frontal, sagittal or any other plane. Such imaging clearly shows the proximal and distal extent of the tumor as well as its relation to surrounding structures (Figs. 7.10 and 7.14). For evaluation of the extent of soft tissue tumors and the extraosseous component of bone tumors with accurate determination of compartmentalization, MRI is clearly superior to any other modality.

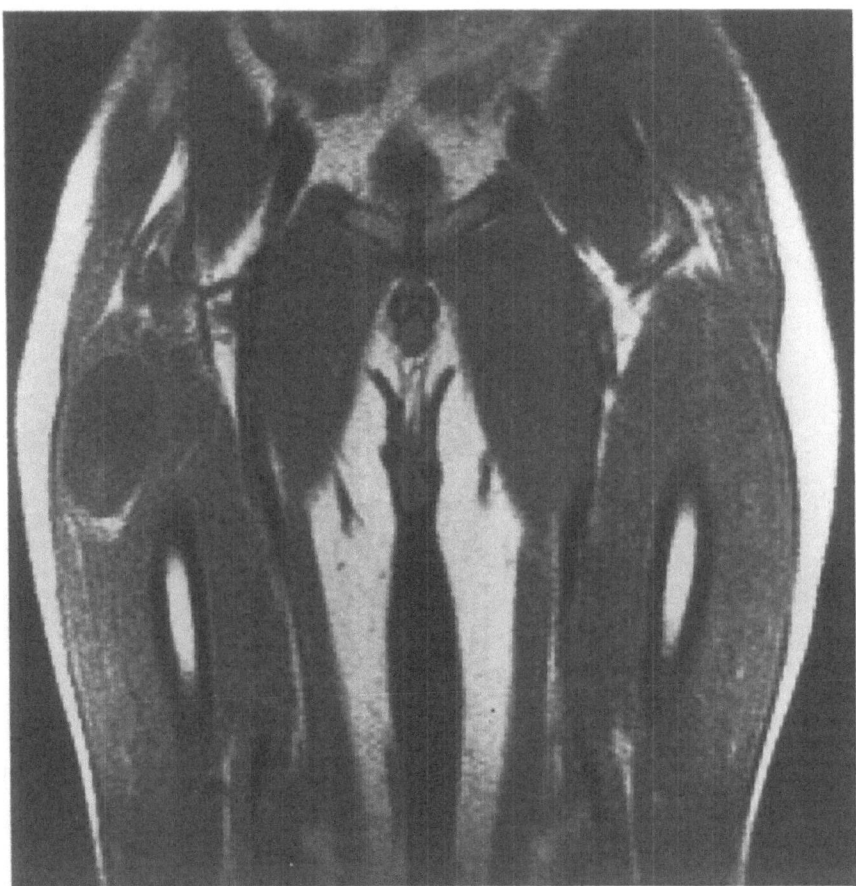

Fig. 7.10. Longitudinal extension of tumor: MRI. Male, 45 years, neurofibroma. SE 500/30 ms, frontal section. The extent of the tumor is clearly outlined, as is the relation between the tumor and the deep fascia.

Involvement of the Neurovascular Bundle

The relationship of the lesion to the major neurovascular bundle is often crucial for the patient, as in many cases this determines whether limb-salvaging resection can be safely performed. Involvement of the neurovascular bundle is present only when there is no normal tissue between the tumor and the vessel. Therefore, the neurovascular bundle may be severely displaced but still not involved. Until the advent of CT, angiography was the only method available for assessment of such involvement.

Angiography is an accurate method for evaluation of the relation between the tumor and the great vessels. The best information is gained in the early arterial phase when contrast medium is shunted over to the neovasculature in the reactive zone around the lesion but still remains in the main arteries also (Fig. 7.11a) (Enneking 1983).

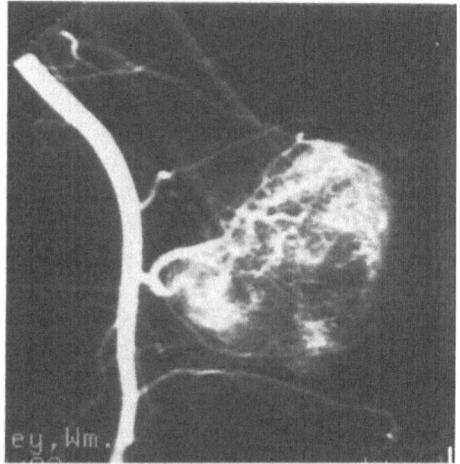

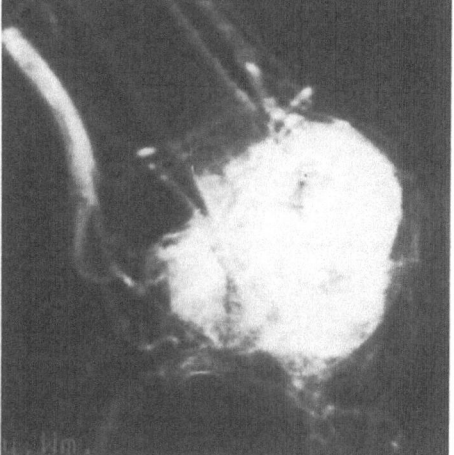

Fig. 7.11a,b. Relation between tumor and the great vessels: angiography. Male, 22 years, osteogenic sarcoma of the distal femur. **a** In the early arterial phase there is contrast medium in the neovasculature of the reactive zone of the tumor, in the femoral and popliteal arteries and in the feeding vessels, clearly revealing the space between the tumor and the main vessels. **b** In the venous phase the draining veins are depicted.

The angiographic examination provides important information also on local blood supply to the tumor, including variation of the normal anatomy, that may be important for planning of the surgery and/or administration of intra-arterial chemotherapy. Information on the degree of hypervascularity may help in the preoperative estimation of possible blood loss, and the vascular pattern will also form the basis for the decision about whether preoperative embolization is demanded. In the venous phase the filling of the draining veins is of value in showing where to apply clamps during surgery to avoid tumor embolization (Enneking 1983) (Fig. 7.11b).

Direct *venography* with injection of contrast medium into the peripheral veins may at times give additional information not only on the anatomic outline and possible dislocation caused by the tumor, but also on tumor growth into the veins. This has been of value in the assessment of, for instance, leiomyosarcomas.

During recent years angiography has been partly replaced by *computed tomography* for assessing involvement of the neurovascular bundle. With contrast-enhanced high-resolution CT information on the relation between the great vessels and the tumor is available in most cases (Heelan et al. 1979; Rosenthal 1985) (Fig. 7.12). However, this plane of normal tissue between the vessel and the tumor may at times be impossible to assess with CT, and in such cases angiography or MRI may give additional information (Fig. 7.13). In tumors extending into the popliteal fossa, the popliteal artery may appear to be situated immediately adjacent to the tumor when the knee is in extension, as it must be during CT examination, while in fact the artery may be totally free from the tumor, as is easily demonstrated at angiography in flexion (Hudson et al. 1983b). The vessel may also be difficult to examine by CT examination in certain anatomic areas, for instance the axillary region (Rosenthal 1982). Thus in selected situations angiography must be performed as well as CT in order to gain sufficient information.

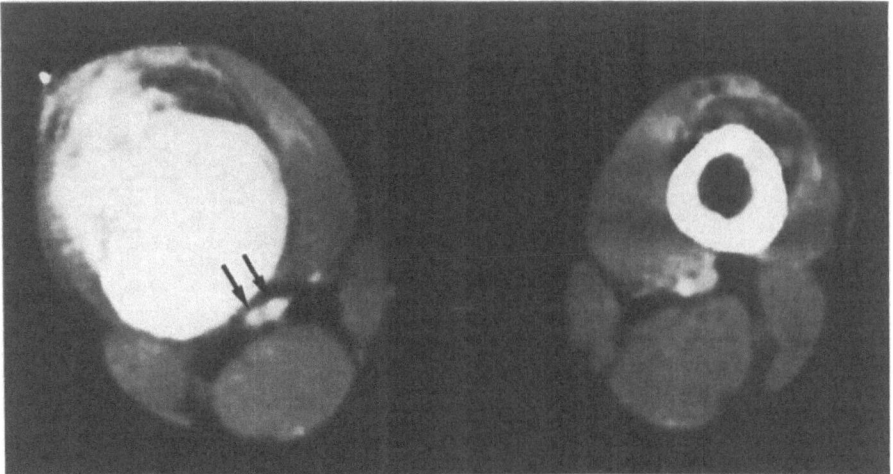

Fig. 7.12. Relation between the tumor and the neurovascular bundle: CT. Male, 10 years, osteogenic sarcoma of the femur. In the transaxial section the contrast-filled femoral artery and vein (*arrows*) are very near the tumor, but there is a thin layer of fat between the tumor and the vessels.

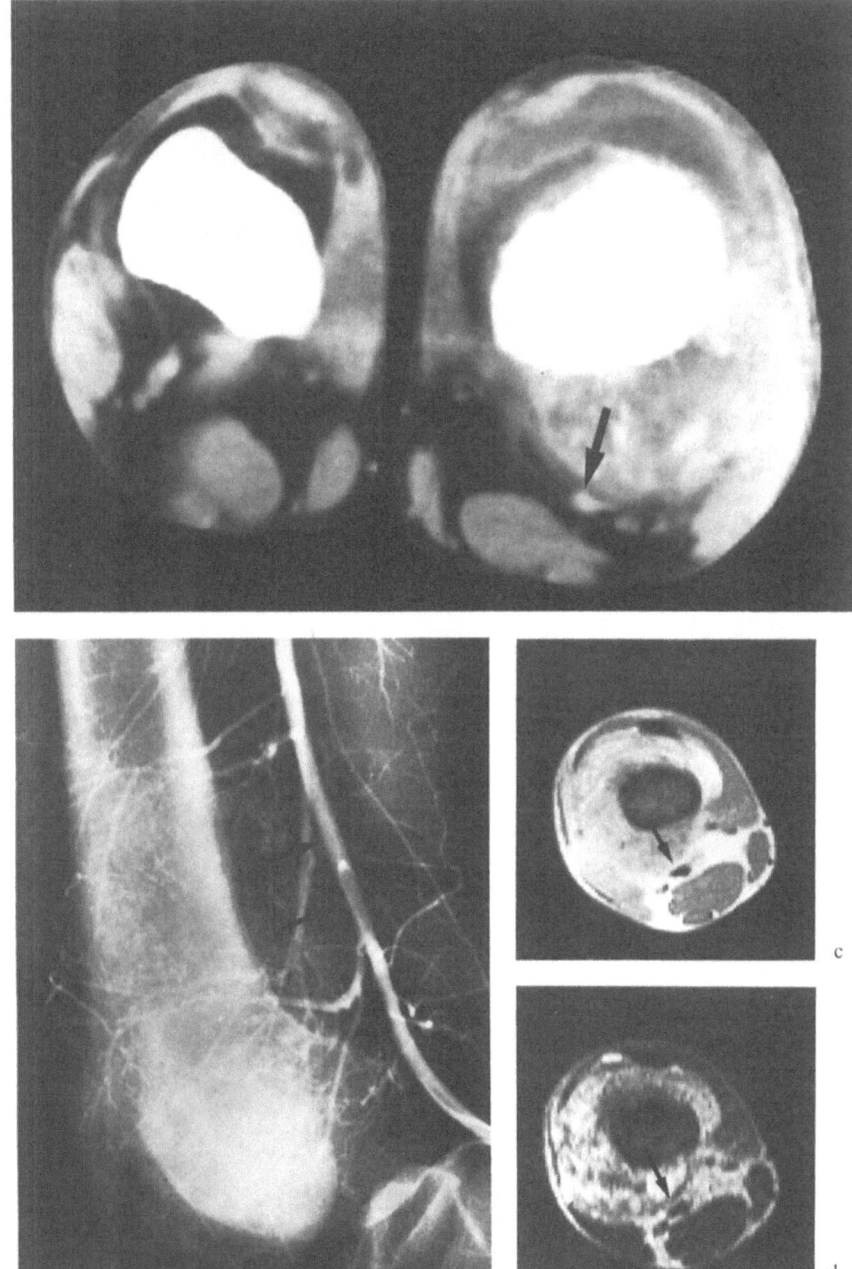

Fig. 7.13a–d. Relation between the neurovascular bundle and the tumor: CT, angiography and MRI. Male, 21 years, osteogenic sarcoma. **a** At the CT examination the femoral artery (*arrow*) is projected immediately adjacent to the tumor, without any obvious normal tissue between the tumor and the vessel. **b** Angiography reveals a very thin strand of tissue between the artery and the hypervascular margin of the tumor (*arrows*). **c** and **d** MRI, SE 500/30 ms (T1-weighted) and 2000/90 ms (T2-weighted), shows clearly a thin layer of fatty tissue between the margin of the tumor and the vessel (*arrow*).

Magnetic resonance imaging has proved to be superior to CT in evaluation of the neurovascular bundle, mainly because it enables study of the vessels in different planes (Fig. 7.14) and because of its high contrast differentiation. Due to the rapid flow in the arteries there is no nuclear magnetic resonance signal from the blood, which therefore appears black and is easy to depict in the image. This has meant considerably decreased use of angiography in centers where MRI is routinely performed (Pettersson et al. 1985a). There are still cases, however, where sufficient information cannot be obtained by MRI—for instance those involving the axillary region. Angiography will then be the ultimate examination.

The nerves are poorly visualized with all available modalities. With good-quality CT examinations the sciatic nerve may be seen at the level of the ischial tuberosity and possibly in the thigh (Fig. 7.7a). The same is true for good-quality MRI images (Fig. 7.7b). With the increased spatial resolution and contrast discrimination provided by new generations of MRI equipment, the possibility of depicting the nerves accurately will increase, which in turn will mean greater potential for precise evaluation of the relationship between a tumor and large nerves as well as its anatomic separation from the big vessels.

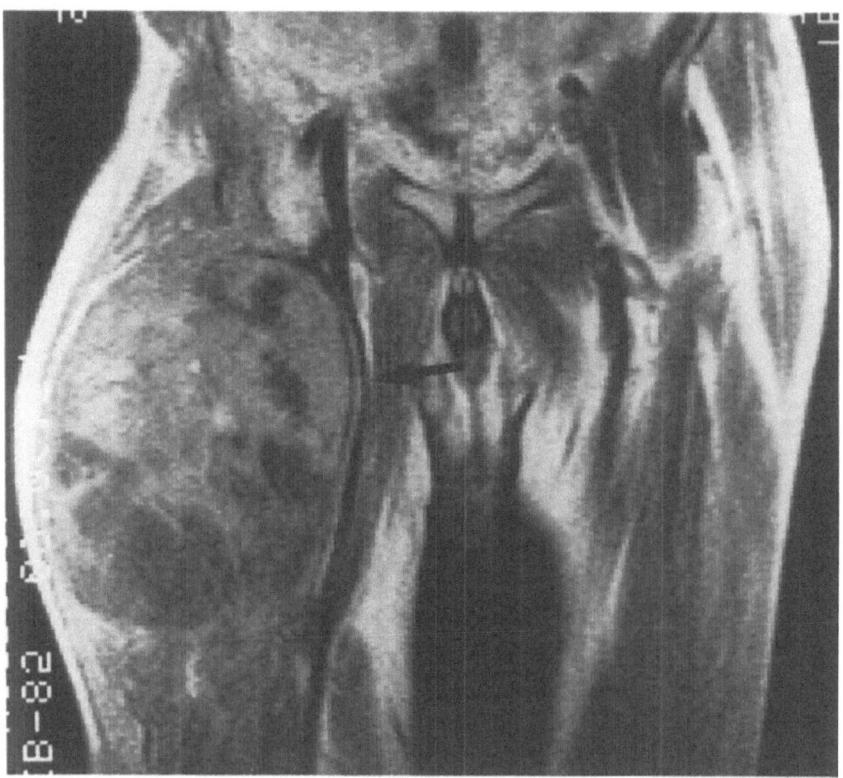

Fig. 7.14. Relation between the artery and the tumor: MRI. Male, 81 years, giant cell soft part sarcoma. MRI, SE 500/30 ms, frontal section, reveals not only the longitudinal extent of the tumor, but also how the femoral artery (*arrow*) is tapered along the medial aspect of the lesion. (From Pettersson et al. 1985, with permission.)

Involvement of Adjacent Bone

A soft tissue malignancy may be in direct contact with an adjacent bone, or there may be invasion of the bone by the tumor, with destruction of the cortex and periosteal reaction. But, from a surgical point of view, it is equally important to determine whether the reactive zone around the tumor is in direct contact with the periosteum, since this necessitates resection of the adjacent bone (Enneking et al. 1981).

On *plain films* cortical erosion and/or periosteal reaction suggesting advanced disease (Fig. 5.17) are only seldom seen. Plain film examination is therefore of limited value.

Scintigraphy with ^{99m}Tc-labelled phosphates or phosphonates has been used as a sensitive technique for depicting radiographically occult bone involvement (Enneking et al. 1981; Hudson et al. 1984b; Kirchner and Simon 1984). Such involvement is present when there is increased uptake in both the tumor and the bone (Fig. 7.15), or when the increased uptake in the tumor is confluent with the activity in the adjacent bone. When there is an area of soft tissue with normal activity between the adjacent bone and the tumor, the bone is not involved (Hudson et al. 1984a) (Figs. 7.16, 7.17). It should be stressed that examination with only whole body images is inadequate: high-resolution target images should be obtained in different planes to explore the bone–tumor relationship tangentially (Fig. 7.18). Using such a technique Hudson et al. (1984a) have achieved a very high accuracy, with virtually no false positive or false negative results.

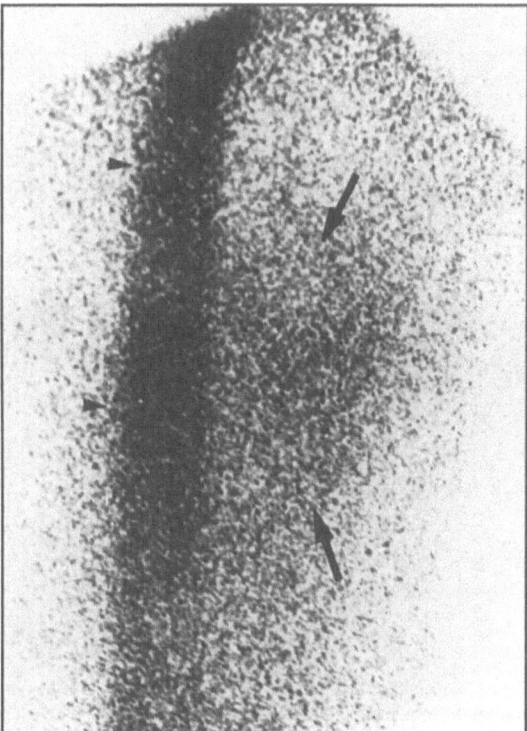

Fig. 7.15. Bone involvement of soft tissue tumor: scintigraphy. Male, 72 years, fibrosarcoma of the thigh. The increased uptake in both the soft tissue tumor (*arrows*) and the femur (*arrowheads*) reveals the bone involvement.

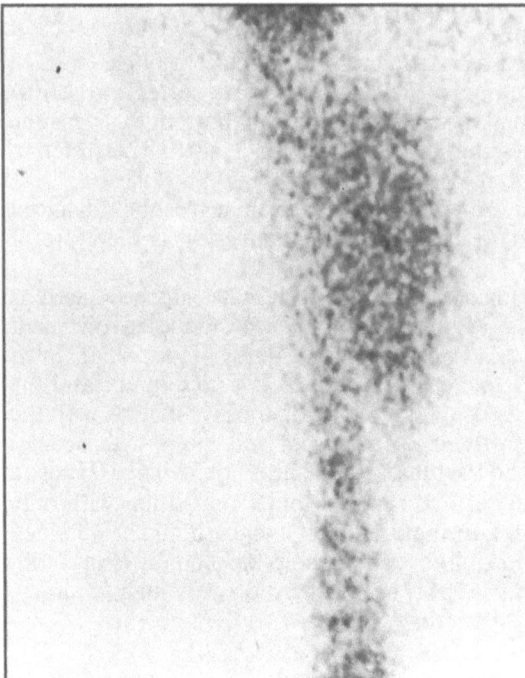

Fig. 7.16. Relation between soft tissue tumor and bone: scintigraphy. Female, 18 years, neurofibroma of the thigh. If the increased uptake in the tumor cannot be separated from the normal uptake of the bone, the bone must be regarded as involved.

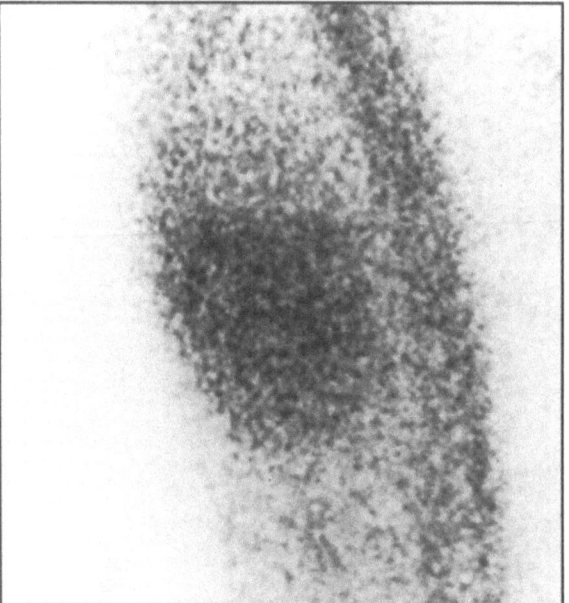

Fig. 17.17. Relation between soft tissue tumor and adjacent bone: scintigraphy. Male, 84 years, malignant fibrous histiocytoma of the thigh. There is an area of soft tissue with normal uptake between the pathologic uptake in the tumor and the normal uptake in the bone. Thus, there is no involvement of the bone.

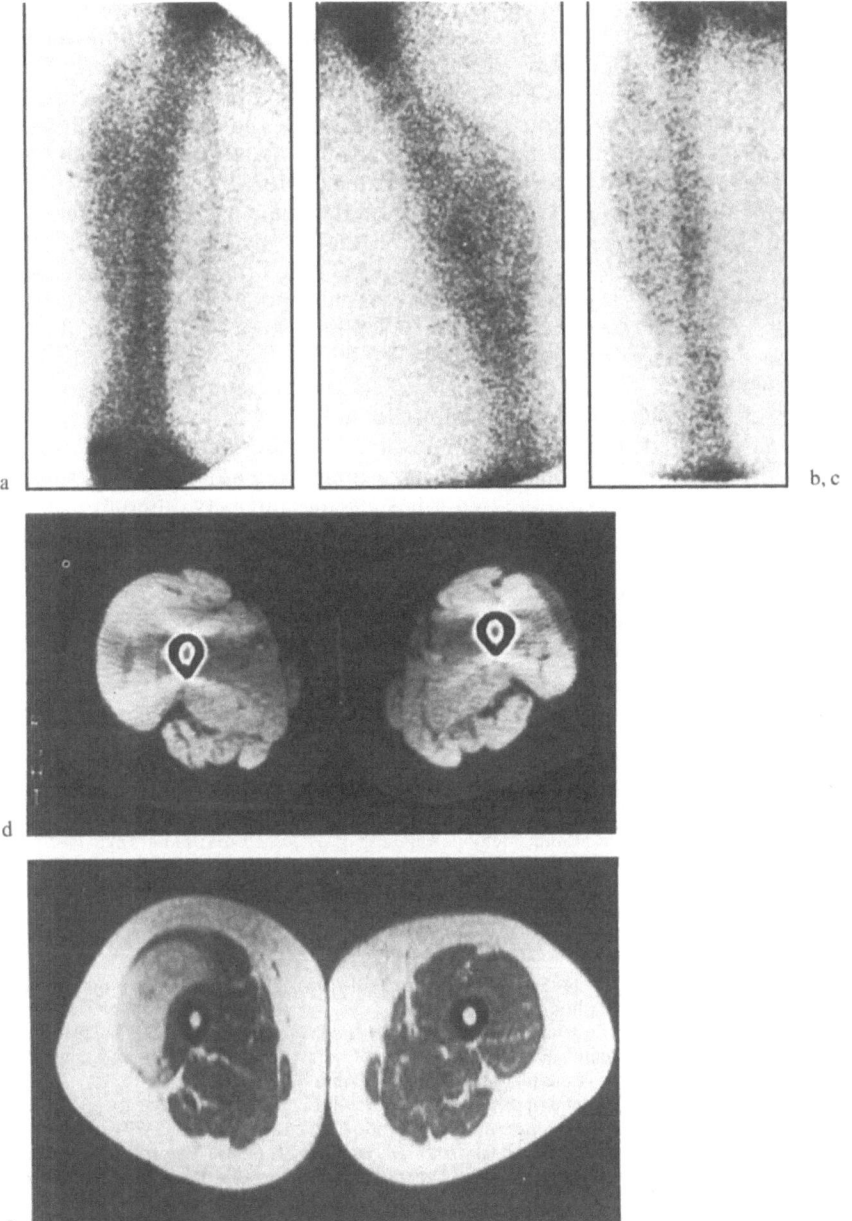

Fig. 7.18a–e. Relation between soft tissue tumor and bone: scintigraphy, CT, and MRI. Female, 54 years, malignant fibrous histiocytoma. **a–c** In the AP (**a**) and lateral (**b**) scintigraphic projections the uptake in the tumor cannot be separated from that in the femur, while in the 20° oblique projection (**c**) there is a strand of tissue with normal uptake between the tumor and the bone. **d** In the CT examination the tumor in the lateral vastus muscle cannot be delineated for several reasons: the attenuation of the tumor is about the same as that of the surrounding muscle, there may be edema and pressure effects at the margins of the tumor, and there are pronounced bone artifacts from the femur. **e** MRI (SE, 2000/30 ms) clearly reveals the tumor and its relation to the femur.

Although *computed tomography* provides a very good evaluation of the extent and relationship of soft tissue tumors, it has pitfalls in the detection of the relationship between soft tissue and bone (deSantos et al. 1979; Heelan et al. 1979; Levine et al. 1979; Egund et al. 1981; Ekelund et al. 1982; Golding and Husband 1982). If a zone of normal tissue is found between the lesion and the adjacent bone, no involvement is present. But, if tumor seems to be immediately adjacent to the bone, this may lead to an overestimation of tumor extent, for many reasons. Edema surrounding the tumor may not be discernible from the lesion itself, or the attenuation value of the tissue may differ very little from that of muscle (Fig. 7.18d) (Jones and Kuhns 1981; Ekelund et al. 1982). In patients with little fat, the CT definition of intramuscular planes is poor. The resolution is also poor in the distal extremities because of their small size and lack of fat (Rosenthal 1982). Furthermore, the bone artifacts seen with most CT machines may diminish the information in the image considerably (Fig. 7.18d). Therefore, in all cases where the CT image is not absolutely clear, the results of scintigraphy should be very helpful.

Magnetic resonance imaging has a substantially better potential than CT for revealing the anatomic relationship between a tumor and adjacent bone, since the inflammatory reaction around the tumor has a signal intensity different from that of the tumor itself and there are no bone artifacts. We have found it as good as scintigraphy in many cases (Pettersson et al. 1985a) (Figs. 7.8b and 7.18e), but the spatial resolution still needs to be improved in most systems in use today. Scintigraphy therefore remains the better technique, particularly in the distal extremities and in children and small adults.

References

Brady TJ, Rosen BR, Pykett IL, McGuire MH, Mankin HJ, Rosenthal DI (1983) NMR imaging of leg tumors. Radiology 149: 181–187

Chew FS, Hudson TM (1982) Radionuclide bone scanning of osteosarcoma: Falsely extended uptake patterns. AJR 139: 49–54

deSantos LA, Goldstein HM, Murray JA, Wallace S (1979) Computed tomography in the evaluation of musculoskeletal neoplasms. Radiology 128: 89–94

DeSmet AA, Neff JR (1982) Knee arthrography for the preoperative evaluation of juxtaarticular masses. Radiology 143: 663–666

DeSmet AA, Levine E, Neff JR (1985) Tumor involvement of peripheral joints other than the knee: Arthrographic evaluation. Radiology 156: 577–601

Egund N, Ekelund L, Sako M, Persson B (1981) CT of soft-tissue tumors. AJR 137: 725–729

Ekelund L, Herrlin K, Rydholm A (1982) Comparison of computed tomography and angiography in the evaluation of soft tissue tumors of the extremities. Acta Radiol [Diagn] 23: 15–29

Enneking WF (1983) Musculoskeletal tumor surgery. Churchill Livingstone, Edinburgh, pp 141–168

Enneking WF, Springfield DS (1977) Osteosarcoma. Orthop Clin North Am 8: 785–794

Enneking WF, Chew FS, Springfield DS, Hudson TM, Spanier SS (1981) The role of radionuclide bone-scanning in determining the resectability of soft-tissue sarcomas. J Bone Joint Surg [Am] 63: 249–257

Finkelstein JB (1975) Tomography and angiography in the evaluation of bone lesions. In: MD Anderson Hospital and Tumor Institute. Radiologic and other biophysical methods in tumor diagnosis. Year Book Medical Publishers, Chicago

Golding SJ, Husband JE (1982) The role of computed tomography in the management of soft tissue sarcomas. Br J Radiol 55: 740–747

Goldman AB, Braunstein P (1975) Augmented radioactivity on bone scans of limbs bearing osteosarcomas. J Nucl Med 16: 423–424

Heelan RT, Watson RC, Smith J (1979) Computed tomography of lower extremity tumors. AJR 132: 933–937

Hudson TM, Hawkins IF Jr. (1981) Radiological evaluation of chondroblastoma. Radiology 139: 1–10

Hudson TM, Chew FS, Manaster BJ (1982) Radionuclide bone scanning of medullary chondrosarcoma. AJR 139: 1071–1076

Hudson TM, Manaster BJ, Springfield DS, Hawkins IF, Enneking WF, Spanier SS (1983a) Radiology of medullary chondrosarcoma: Preoperative treatment planning. Skeletal Radiol 10: 69–78

Hudson TM, Schiebler M, Springfield DS, Hawkins IF, Enneking WF, Spanier SS (1983b) Radiologic imaging of osteosarcoma: Role in planning surgical treatment. Skeletal Radiol 10: 137–146

Hudson TM, Schakel M, Springfield DS, Spanier SS, Enneking WF (1984a) The comparative value of bone scintigraphy and computed tomography in determining bone involvement by soft-tissue sarcomas. J Bone Joint Surg [Am] 66: 1400–1407

Hudson TM, Schiebler M, Springfield DS, Enneking WF, Hawkins IF Jr., Spanier SS (1984b) Radiology of giant cell tumors of bone: Computed tomography, arthro-tomography, and scintigraphy. Skeletal Radiol 11: 85–95

Hudson TM, Hamlin DJ, Enneking WF, Pettersson H (1985) Magnetic resonance imaging of bone and soft tissue tumors: Early experience in 31 patients compared with computed tomography. Skeletal Radiol 13: 134–146

Jones ET, Kuhns LR (1981) Pitfalls in the use of computed tomography for musculoskeletal tumors in children. J Bone Joint Surg [Am] 63: 1297–1304

Kirchner PT, Simon MA (1984) The clinical value of bone and gallium scintigraphy for soft-tissue sarcomas of the extremities. J Bone Joint Surg [Am] 66: 319–327

Levine E, Lee KR, Neff JR, Maklad MF, Robinson RG, Preston DF (1979) Comparison of computed tomography and other imaging modalities in the evaluation of musculoskeletal tumors. Radiology 131: 431–437

Moon KL, Davis PL, Kaufman L et al. (1983) Nuclear magnetic resonance imaging of a fibrosarcoma tumor implanted in the rat. Radiology 148: 177–181

Pettersson H, Hamlin DJ, Enneking WF, Springfield DS, Andrew ER, Spanier S, Slone R (1985a) MR imaging of primary musculoskeletal tumors: Experience from 193 examinations. Radiology 157(P): 109

Pettersson H, Hamlin DJ, Mancuso A, Scott KN (1985b) Magnetic resonance imaging of the musculoskeletal system. Acta Radiol 25: 225–235

Reiser M, Rupp N, Heller H-J, Allgayer B, Lukas P, Lange J, Pfafferott K, Fink U (1984) MR-tomography in the diagnosis of malignant soft-tissue tumors. Eur J Radiol 4: 288–293

Rosenthal DI (1982) Computed tomography in bone and soft tissue neoplasm: Application and pathologic correlation. CRC Crit Rev Diagn Imaging 18: 243–277

Rosenthal DI (1985) Computed tomography of orthopedic neoplasms. Orthop Clin North Am 16: 461–470

Simon MA, Kirchner PT (1980) Scintigraphic evaluation of primary bone tumors. J Bone Joint Surg [Am] 62: 758–764

Soye I, Levine E, DeSmet AA, Neff JR (1982) Computed tomography in the preoperative evaluation of masses arising in or near the joints of the extremities. Radiology 143: 727–732

Springfield DS, Enneking WF, Neff JR, Mahley JT (1984) Principles of tumor management. In: Murray JA (ed) AAOS instructional course lectures. CV Mosby, St. Louis, pp 1–25

Thrall JH, Geslien GE, Corcoran RJ, Johnson MC (1975) Abnormal radionuclide deposition patterns adjacent to focal skeletal lesions. Radiology 115: 659–663

Watts HG (1980) Introduction to resection of musculoskeletal sarcomas. Clin Orthop 153: 31–38

Wilner D (1982) Radiology of bone tumors and allied disorders. WB Saunders, Philadelphia, pp 25–75

Zimmer WD, Berquist TH, McLeod RA et al. (1985) Bone tumors: Magnetic resonance imaging versus computed tomography. Radiology 155: 709–718

Chapter 8

Radiologic Appearance of the Response to Treatment

Surgery, radiation therapy, and chemotherapy each produce a distinctive response within the lesion and in the surrounding tissue that may be evaluated with diagnostic imaging techniques.

Surgery

An incision through the reactive zone and capsule into the lesion, whether deliberate as in incisional biopsy or inadvertent during attempts to excise a lesion, contaminates all of the tissues exposed by the incision. Cells within the lesion may potentially be transplanted anywhere in the exposed tissues and may produce local extension and/or local recurrences. Hemorrhage from within the lesion, whether as a result of incisional biopsy, incomplete excision or blunt trauma, may not only contaminate tissue planes exposed by the incision but may also spread more extensively along undissected tissue planes and produce more widespread contamination (Springfield et al. 1984).

Following excision of a lesion the wound fills with blood which quickly becomes organized and replaced by granulation tissue. The granulation tissue in turn matures into reactive mesenchymal tissue and differentiates into either bone (if within the skeleton) or fibrous tissue (if in the soft tissues). This reparative response reaches its zenith in 10–14 days and gradually abates over the next 3–4 weeks. For this reason, all diagnostic imaging needed for planning of the definitive surgery should be done, whenever possible and practicable, prior to biopsy. If done after biopsy, the reparative response to the biopsy may often obscure or cause misinterpretation of the radiologic studies.

In the bone, the cavity resulting from the biopsy should pose no difficulty in the interpretation of the plain films; however, all radiologic studies, including scintigraphy, angiography and CT, are more difficult to interpret after biopsy (Simon 1982). In the bone, increased isotope uptake can be mistaken for evidence of tumor, as can vascular granulation tissue at angiography. In the soft tissue, edema, hemorrhage and inflammatory changes may already be difficult or impossible to distinguish from tumor with any modality, including CT, before surgery (Jones and

Kuhns 1980; Egund et al. 1981; Ekelund et al. 1982), and these difficulties are enhanced after surgical intervention. Hudson et al. (1985) have shown that in patients who had had prior surgical biopsy, CT could not correctly predict the presence or absence of microscopic residual tumor and was inaccurate in distinguishing tumor from scar tissue.

MRI, with its better soft tissue contrast resolution and better possibilities for tissue characterization, should have a greater potential in post-biopsy evaluation than CT, but no reports on this are on record. In our experience it has been possible in some cases to distinguish inflammatory reaction and hemorrhage from residual tumor; when the inflammatory reaction has subsided and only a fibrotic scar remains, such tissue can be distinguished from tumor by its low signal intensity (Pettersson et al. 1985). However, in several cases we have been unable to distinguish by MRI the reaction after biopsy from residual tumor.

When microscopic residual tumor is left in a wound, the reparative response to the surgical procedure overwhelms the neoplastic cells and obscures them from even microscopic detection until the wound matures. Microscopic residual disease usually does not become histologically evident for at least 6–8 weeks afterwards and more often 3–4 months. Thus, if microscopic residual tumor has been documented histologically following incomplete removal or excisional biopsy, subsequent staging to ascertain its extent should, when practicable, be postponed until the mesenchymal response to the procedure has abated.

Following an incisional or excisional biopsy, accurate identification of the tissue planes contaminated by the biopsy may be of key importance in planning the definitive surgical procedure or mapping out radiation fields. MRI is the best method for this. Even if it is not always possible to distinguish the reparative reactive tissue from residual neoplastic tissue, MRI will quite accurately distinguish either of these abnormalities from normal tissue.

Radiation Therapy

Radiation therapy produces patchy areas of necrosis in and around which dense acellular fibrillar material replaces the lesional tissue. These areas of necrosis are histologically evident as early as 2 weeks after completion of the therapy. The extent of the necrosis depends upon the amount and timing of the radiation energy and the responsiveness or sensitivity of the lesion to the therapy. Wide variation occurs from lesion to lesion and patient to patient.

Perhaps more important surgically, however, is the development of a thick, dense, fibrous capsule around the lesion. This zone of acellular collagenized fibrous tissue replaces the immature proliferating reactive zone that forms the pseudocapsule, and often appears to obliterate the satellites in the reactive zone. When effective, radiation therapy appears to convert the thick, reactive pseudocapsule around a soft tissue sarcoma into a tough, dense "rind" that makes dissection from surrounding normal tissue easier than in an untreated lesion.

The effects of radiation therapy in bone and bone marrow are dependent upon the age of the patient, the anatomic structure irradiated and its physiological state before treatment, the extent of irradiated tissue, the radiation dose, the pattern of application and the use of radiation modifiers (Parker and Berry 1976). The clinical sequence of changes may be divided into four periods: (1) acute (first 6 months); (2) subacute (6–12 months); (3) chronic (1–5 years); late (more than 5 years). The radiologic changes recorded would thus vary with the time elapsed since the treatment, and they would also be heavily dependent on the type of tumor irradiated (Wilner 1982). Any detailed discussion of the post-radiation changes is outside the scope of this book, but some principles should be stressed.

During and after radiation therapy, diagnostic imaging can accurately document the skeletal extent and appearance of diseased tissue, volumetric change in the lesion, and the relationship of the tumor to the adjacent fascial planes and neurovascular bundles. But for results to be comparable it is absolutely mandatory that when the imaging is repeated, identical examination techniques are used. Thus, plain film examinations must be made in exactly the same projection, isotope scans repeated in comparable planes, CT sections done at comparable levels with consistent window settings, and MRI images reconstructed with identifiable landmarks. The post-radiation diagnostic imaging may be crucial to the decision of whether to proceed with a limb-salvaging excision or an amputation; but they are of limited value when done haphazardly and without careful review of the initial pre-treatment studies.

Chemotherapy

The biologic response to chemotherapy is a coagulative type of necrosis that usually appears in a responsive lesion within 2 weeks of the third or fourth cycle of the drug therapy. A histologic grading system has been devised based on the proportion of necrosis to viable tissue as follows: 1, 0–10% necrosis; 2, 10%–50% necrosis; 3, 50%–90% necrosis; 4, more than 90% necrosis. This system has proved valuable in quantifying the response to chemotherapy, in planning the extent of subsequent definitive surgical procedures, and in guiding further drug therapy.

Several attempts have been made to monitor tumor response radiologically, and good correlation has been claimed between the histologic response and the plain film radiography (Chuang et al. 1982; Smith et al. 1982), scintigraphy (Goldstein et al. 1980), angiography (Chuang et al. 1982; Jaffe et al. 1983) and CT (Mail et al. 1985; Shirkhoda et al. 1985). The decrease in soft tissue swelling can be appreciated by most methods. In the tumor matrix of osteosarcomas, two types of calcification occur, one peripheral and the other central. These are best seen by plain film radiography and CT. The change of bone structure to a more mature pattern is best seen by plain film radiography. Quantification of the disappearance of tumor vascularity as seen by angiography correlates well with the histologic response (Chuang et al. 1982; Jaffe et al. 1983). MRI should have a great potential for recording tumor response, but so far only a few encouraging reports are on record (Mancuso et al. 1984).

Accurate grading of the response to chemotherapy still requires excision of a significant portion of the lesion, and non-invasive radiographic imaging has yet to offer comparable accuracy. When available, such non-invasive quantification techniques will be extremely valuable.

References

Chuang VP, Benjamin R, Jaffe N et al. (1982) Radiographic and angiographic changes in osteosarcoma after intraarterial chemotherapy. AJR 139: 1065–1069

Egund N, Ekelund L, Sako M, Persson B (1981) CT of soft-tissue tumors. AJR 137: 725–729

Ekelund L, Herrlin K, Rydholm A (1982) Comparison of computed tomography and angiography in the evaluation of soft tissue tumors of the extremities. Acta Radiol [Diagn] 23: 15–28

Goldstein H, McNeil BJ, Zufall E, Jaffe MB, Treves S (1980) Changing indications for bone scintigraphy in patients with osteosarcoma. Radiology 135: 177–180

Hudson TM, Schakel M II, Springfield DS (1985) Limitations of computed tomography following excisional biopsy of soft tissue sarcomas. Skeletal Radiol 13: 49–54

Jaffe N, Knapp J, Chuang VP et al. (1983) Osteosarcoma: Intra-arterial treatment of the primary tumor with cis-diamminedichloroplatinum II (CDD). Cancer 51: 402–407

Jones ET, Kuhns LR (1980) Pitfalls in the use of computed tomography for musculoskeletal tumors in children. J Bone Joint Surg [Am] 63: 1277–1304

Mail JT, Cohen MD, Mirkin LD, Provisor AJ (1985) Response of osteosarcoma to preoperative intravenous high-dose methotrexate chemotherapy: CT evaluation. AJR 144: 89–93

Mancuso A, Fitzsimmons J, Mareci I, Million R, Cassisi N (1984) MR imaging of the upper pharynx and neck. Variations of normal and possible applications in detecting and staging malignant tumors. II. Pathology. Radiology 153(P): 140

Parker RG, Berry HC (1976) Late effects of therapeutic irradiation on the skeleton and bone marrow. Cancer 37: 1162–1172

Pettersson H, Hamlin DJ, Enneking WF, Springfield DS, Andrew ER, Spanier S, Slone R (1985) MR imaging of primary musculoskeletal tumors: Experience from 193 examinations. Radiology 157(P): 109

Shirkhoda A, Jaffe N, Wallace S, Ayala A, Lindell MM, Zornoza J (1985) Computed tomography of osteosarcoma after intraarterial chemotherapy. AJR 144: 95–99

Simon MA (1982) Biopsy of musculoskeletal tumors. J Bone Joint Surg [Am] 64: 1253–1257

Smith J, Heelan RT, Huvos AG et al. (1982) Radiographic changes in primary osteogenic sarcoma following intensive chemotherapy. Radiology 143: 355–360

Springfield DS, Enneking WF, Neff JR, Mahley JT (1984) Principles of tumor management. In: Murray JA (ed) AAOS instructional course lectures. CV Mosby, St. Louis, pp 1–24

Wilner D (1982) Radiology of bone tumors and allied disorders. WB Saunders, Philadelphia, pp 25–75

Chapter 9
Imaging Protocols

From the previous chapters it should be clear that the different imaging modalities may provide the same type of information in the investigation of musculoskeletal tumors, while in several important aspects they complement each other. A total diagnostic work-up is expensive and may be inconvenient and tiresome for the patient. Therefore, protocols should be sought that give optimal information with as few examinations as possible.

The Relative Values of the Different Imaging Modalities

In an attempt to examine the relative importance of the different imaging modalities, we reviewed 121 examinations of bone and soft tissue tumors (Pettersson et al. 1985). The following tumors were included: aneurysmal bone cyst (5 patients), giant cell tumor (15), osteosarcoma (25), chondrosarcoma (13), lipoma (8), fibromatosis (10), liposarcoma (16), and malignant fibrous histiocytoma (29). Plain films were available in 90% of the patients, angiography in 27%, scintigraphy in 75%, CT in 95%, and MRI in 100%. The histology and surgical findings were known in all patients. In our review each of the following parameters was evaluated for each patient and each examination: intraosseous extension; extraosseous extension; cortical destruction; calcification and ossification within and around the tumor; periosteal/endosteal reaction; delineation between tumor and muscle, tumor and vessel, tumor and fat, tumor and nerve, tumor and joint, tumor and necrosis/bleeding; as well as bone involvement of soft tissue tumors. A score was given to each examination according to the information available in the image as compared with the known histologic and surgical findings. Possible scores ranged from 5 to 1: 5 = excellent, 4 = good, 3 = fair, 2 = poor, 1 = not evaluable. It should be noted that not all parameters of importance in the diagnostic work-up are included: for example, multiplicity of the tumor, skip lesions, distant metastases in bone and lung metastases were not evaluated.

The findings were compared for each diagnostic group using Dunkin's multiple range procedure. The results for the skeletal part of bone tumors confined to the skeleton are given in Table 9.1. There were no differences found between soft tissue tumors and the soft tissue component of bone tumors with extension outside the bone, and the results for these lesions are presented together in Table 9.2. The tables give the mean score for each modality and parameter, as well as the significance of the difference found between the modalities. It is clear that several of the modalities had similar scores that were not significantly different. Thus, although MRI had the highest score for intraosseous and extraosseous extent of bone tumors (Table 9.1), it was not significantly better than CT for extraosseous extent nor than CT or scintigraphy for intraosseous extent. For soft tissue tumors, and the soft tissue component of bone tumors with cortical breakthrough, MRI was superior in all parameters evaluated, though it was not significantly better than angiography for evaluation of the tumor/vessel relationship nor better than CT for tumor/fat delineation or scintigraphy for evaluation of bone involvement.

Table 9.1. Information value of different imaging modalities: Primary bone tumors

Parameter	MRI	CT	Angiography	Scintigraphy	Plain film
Extraosseous extension	△4.1	△3.6	□2.9	○2.6	○1.7
Intraosseous extension	△4.5	△4.2	○2.9	△4.4	□3.3
Cortical destruction	□3.0	△4.0			△3.6
Calcification, ossification	○1.6	△3.8			□3.0
Periosteal/endosteal reaction	○1.6	□2.1			□3.4

△ is significantly better than □, which in turn is significantly better than ○ (at $P<0.05$).

Table 9.2. Information value of different imaging modalities: Soft tissue tumors and bone tumors with soft tissue extension

Parameter	MRI	CT	Angiography	Scintigraphy	Plain film
Tumor–muscle delineation	△4.3	□3.3	○2.5		
Tumor–vessel delineation	△4.2	□3.1	△4.5		
Tumor–nerve delineation	△1.6	△1.1			
Tumor–fat delineation	△4.4	□3.9			
Bone involvement (soft tissue)	△4.3	□3.5	○2.9	△4.0	○2.2
Tumor–joint delineation	△4.4	□2.9			□2.6
Tumor–necrosis/bleeding delineation	△4.1	□3.1			

△ is significantly better than □, which in turn is significantly better than ○ (at $P<0.05$).

It is obvious that if two methods give the same information, the one that is more easily performed and of less risk for the patient should be chosen. Thus, in the evaluation of the relation between tumor and vessel, for instance, MRI should be used, and only if this method fails should angiography be performed.

Given these results and the experiences discussed in previous chapters, we propose the follow protocols:

Proposed Protocols

Bone Tumors

Bone tumors should be examined first with *plain film*, which supplies a wealth of information on the local behavior of the tumor, diagnosis and local extent. If further examination is needed, the next step should be *scintigraphy*, which gives information on multiplicity of the tumor including skip lesions and bone metastases, as well as bone reaction and intraosseous extent. Further information is provided by *computed tomography*, especially on specific tumor patterns, intraosseous extent and cortical breakthrough. In suspected malignant bone tumor, *plain film chest examination* and *chest CT* should be performed as baseline examinations before surgery. If joint involvement cannot be excluded, MRI should be added and, possibly, arthrography.

Soft Tissue Tumors and Bone Tumors with Soft Tissue Extension

For soft tissue tumors and bone tumors with soft tissue extension, *plain film* examination yields little, but is easily performed with little discomfort to the patient and could be done as an initial survey examination. *Scintigraphy* provides some additional information on the local behavior of the tumor, multiplicity of the lesion and possible involvement of adjacent bone. For all other important information— specific tumor patterns, local extension, involvement of the neurovascular bundle, etc.— *MRI* should be used. CT is not necessary, except for a *chest CT* as a baseline in the search for metastases, and for this a *plain film chest examination* should also be performed. Angiography should be used only if the other methods do not give sufficient information on the relationship betwen the neurovascular bundle and the tumor, or if there is a vascular lesion.

It should be stressed that these protocols are only basic guidelines and that the ultimate choice of modalities must always be determined by the clinical findings and the findings during the examinations. The practical approach in different clinical situations is illustrated by the case examples in Chapter 10.

Reference

Pettersson H, Hamlin DJ, Enneking WF, Springfield DS, Andrew ER, Spanier S, Slone R (1985) MR imaging of musculoskeletal tumors: Experience from 193 examinations. Radiology 157(P): 109

Chapter 10

Case Examples

The following cases were selected to illustrate the radiologic protocols and common findings in both benign and malignant musculoskeletal tumors with varying degrees of aggressiveness. As stated in previous chapters, it is the synthesis of the radiologic findings and all other data that forms the basis for the clinical management. Therefore, these cases should be regarded only as case *examples*. Confronted with the individual patient the radiologist may always adjust the protocols according to previous radiologic and clinical findings, the orthopedic surgeon's needs, his own experience and the equipment available.

Case 1

A 15-year-old female had a sprained knee and on the same day had a plain radiograph taken. One week later she saw the orthopedic surgeon and at that time she was asymptomatic.

The anteroposterior (AP) and lateral radiographs of the distal femur (case 1, Fig. 1a,b) reveal geographic destruction at the metaphyseal cortex on the medial side. There is a narrow transition zone with a cortical capsule around the radiolucency which involves the cortex. There is no evidence of periosteal reaction and no suggestion of a soft tissue mass.

Radiographically this is a latent lesion and both the clinical presentation and the radiographic findings are consistent with a non-ossifying fibroma.

Because the patient's family were quite anxious, scintigraphy was performed (case 1, Fig. 2), which showed no increased uptake of the ^{99m}Tc-labelled nucleotide in the area of the lesion. This confirms that the lesion is latent, and most probably a non-ossifying fibroma. No further diagnostic studies and no treatment are indicated.

Surgical stage: 1.

A follow-up radiograph 3 years later (case 1, Fig. 3) showed resolution of the lesion with slight overhealing.

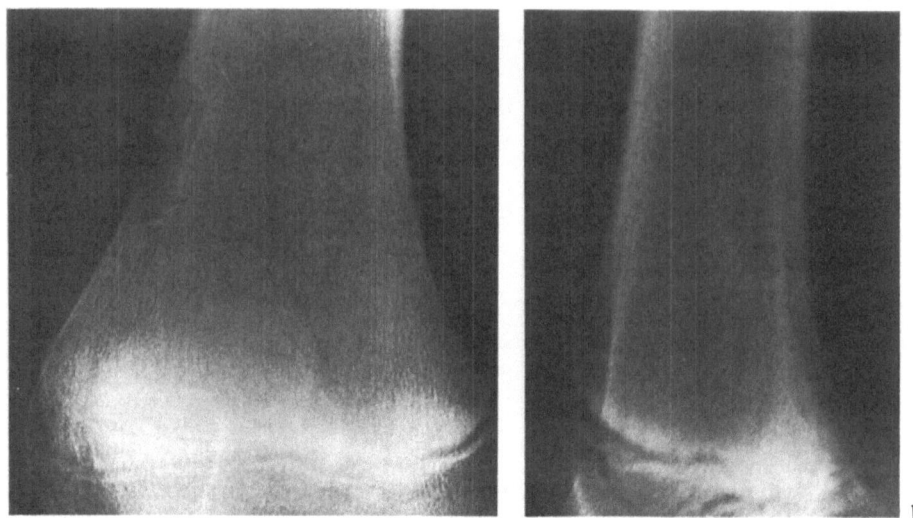

a
b

Fig. 1

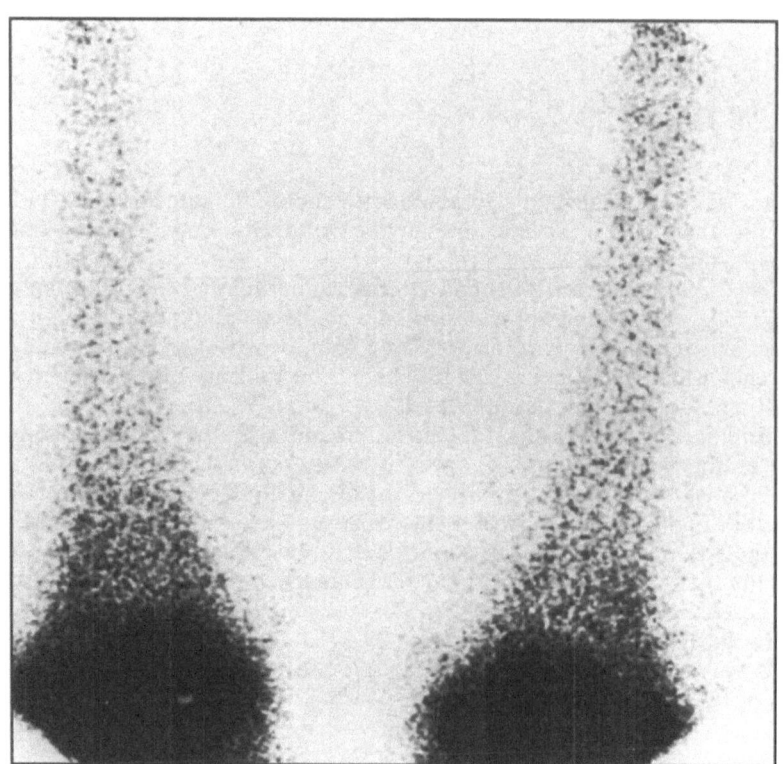

Fig. 2

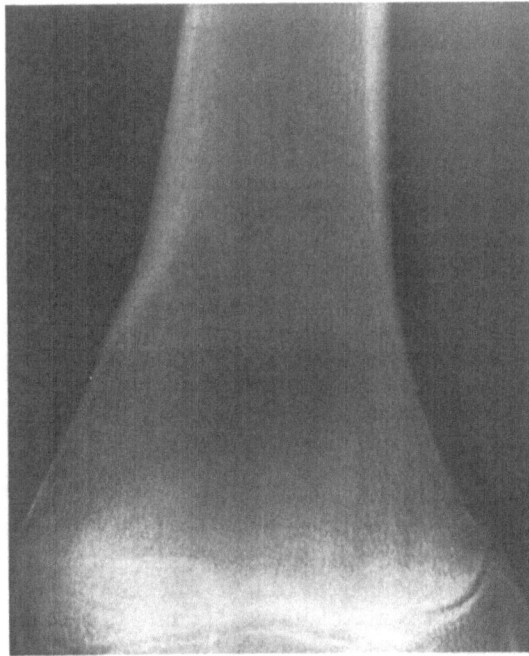

Fig. 3

Case 2

A 25-year-old female presented with a history of knee pain for 1 month. On physical examination there was tenderness over the lateral femoral condyle. There was no swelling and the range of motion was normal.

On the AP radiograph of the knee (case 2, Fig. 1) there is a geographic destruction in the lateral femoral condyle with a narrow transition zone lacking a well-developed reactive rim; the cortex remains intact.

The initial presentation, the clinical history and the physical and radiographic examination are consistent with at least an active tumor; therefore, additional evaluation with scintigraphy and CT is indicated.

Scintigraphy (case 2, Fig. 2a,b) reveals increased uptake of the radionucleotide only in the lateral femoral condyle, the extent of the uptake corresponding with the extent of the lesion as seen on the plain radiograph. Decreased uptake in the center of this lesion is consistent with a giant cell tumor, as is the appearance of the plain radiograph.

This lesion requires treatment and its exact extent must be determined prior to surgery.

The CT examination (case 2, Fig. 3) reveals a destructive lesion within the medullary canal with thinning (but no disruption) of the cortex and soft tissue component. The attenuation values of the lesion were measured on images obtained before and during contrast medium infusion (case 2, Fig. 4a,b). The values rose from 56 HU without intravenous contrast to 104 HU with contrast, which indicates a vascular tumor.

The clinical history, plain radiograph, the scintigraphy and the CT examination, including the enhancement during intravenous infusion of contrast medium, are all consistent with an active lesion, most probably a giant cell tumor of bone.

The patient was treated with an incisional biopsy, extensive curettage and packing with polymethylmethacrylate. The final histologic diagnosis was giant cell tumor of bone.

Surgical stage: 2.

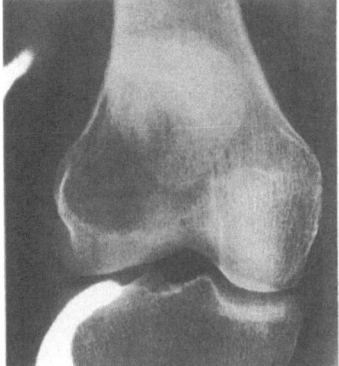

Fig. 1

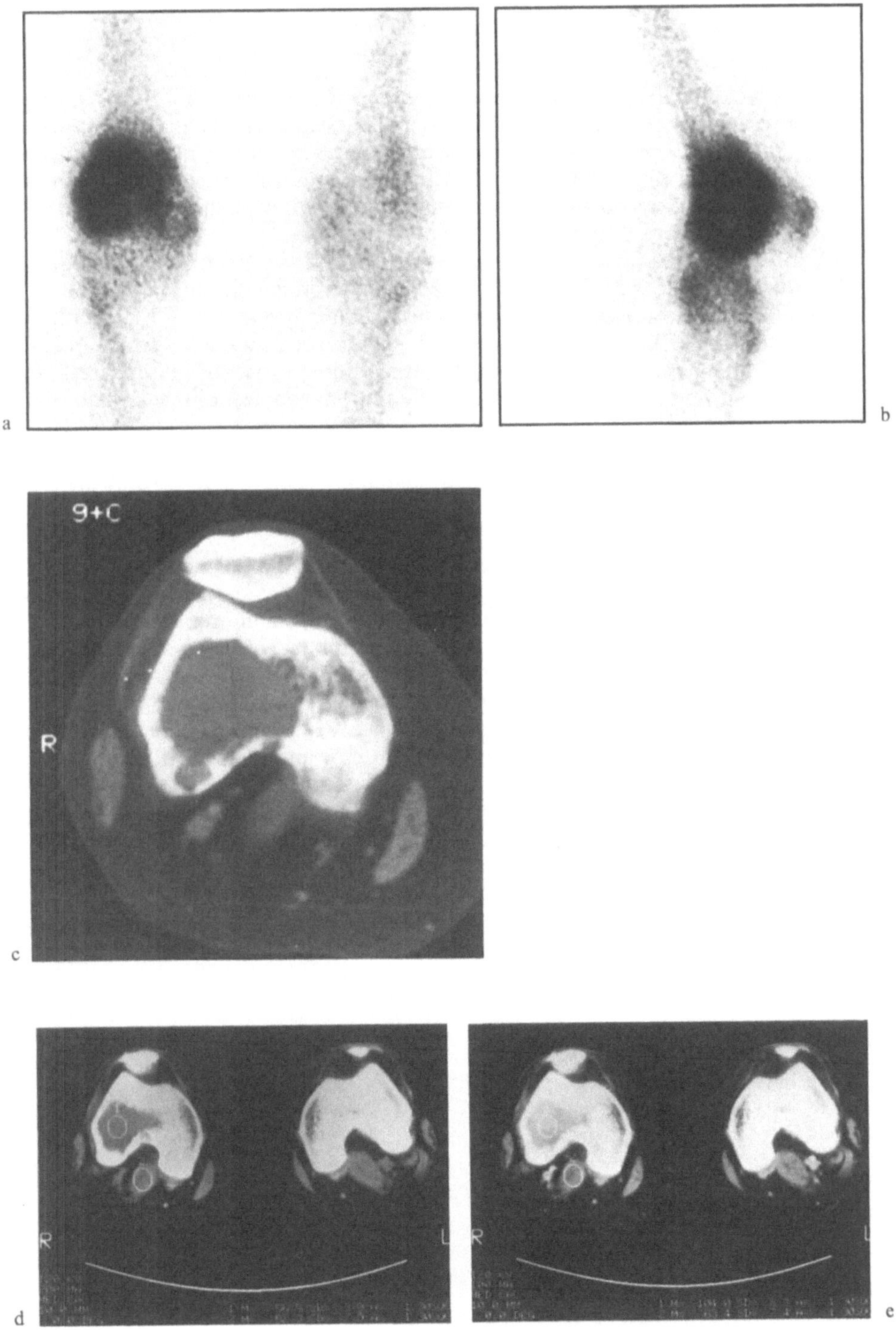

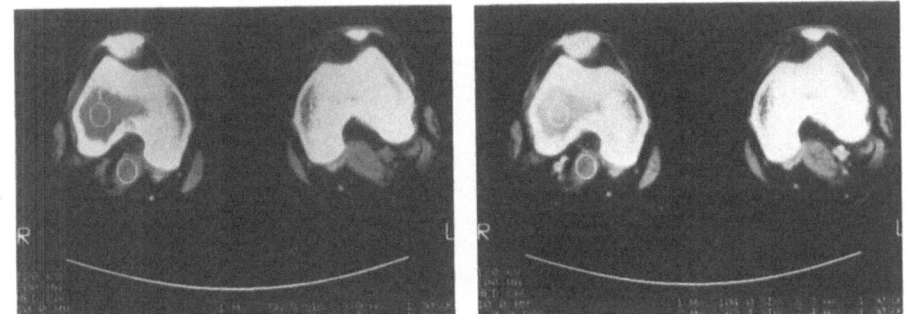

Fig. 2

Case 3

A 20-year-old female had noticed an enlarging tumor in the posterior distal thigh for approximately 3 months. She was otherwise asymptomatic and had no other illness. On physical examination the patient had a large non-tender firm movable mass in the distal thigh and popliteal fossa. She had a full range of motion in her knee and there were no neurologic disturbances. Direct palpation produced a Tinel's sign with radiation down into the posterior ankle.

A soft tissue mass without calcifications is seen on the plain lateral radiograph of the distal thigh (case 3, Fig. 1; arrows). The underlying bone appears normal.

The early phase of scintigraphy (radionuclide angiogram) (case 3, Fig. 2a) shows increased vascularity within the lesion. The delayed scan (case 3, Fig. 2b) reveals increased uptake of the nucleotide within the lesion, particularly in its distal portion. There is no evidence of increased activity in the adjacent bone and no other "hot spots".

In our experience a CT scan of a soft tissue tumor is unnecessary when the lesion is not adjacent to the bone and MRI is available. Therefore a CT scan was not done on this patient.

On the sagittal sections of the MRI examination (case 3, Fig. 3) the lesion is well delineated and homogeneous, except for two small areas with a lower signal intensity consistent with cystic contents (arrows). It has a smooth capsule and appears to be surrounded by normal fat, except in a small area where it may be immediately adjacent to the bone. A structure of similar characteristics to the tumor (arrowhead) at the proximal end of the lesion was interpreted to be the sciatic nerve.

A transverse section of the MRI (case 3, Fig. 4) reveals that the mass does not involve the muscle and appears to be immediately adjacent to bone. In all other transverse sections there was fat between the tumor and the bone. The vessels are immediately adjacent to this mass.

The radiologic chest examination (plain film and CT) was normal.

The clinical presentation and radiographic findings suggest an active lesion possibly arising within the nerve. Only the large size of the lesion is suggestive of a malignancy.

An incisional biopsy revealed a benign neurofibroma and a marginal excision was accomplished without sacrificing the sciatic nerve.

Surgical stage: 2.

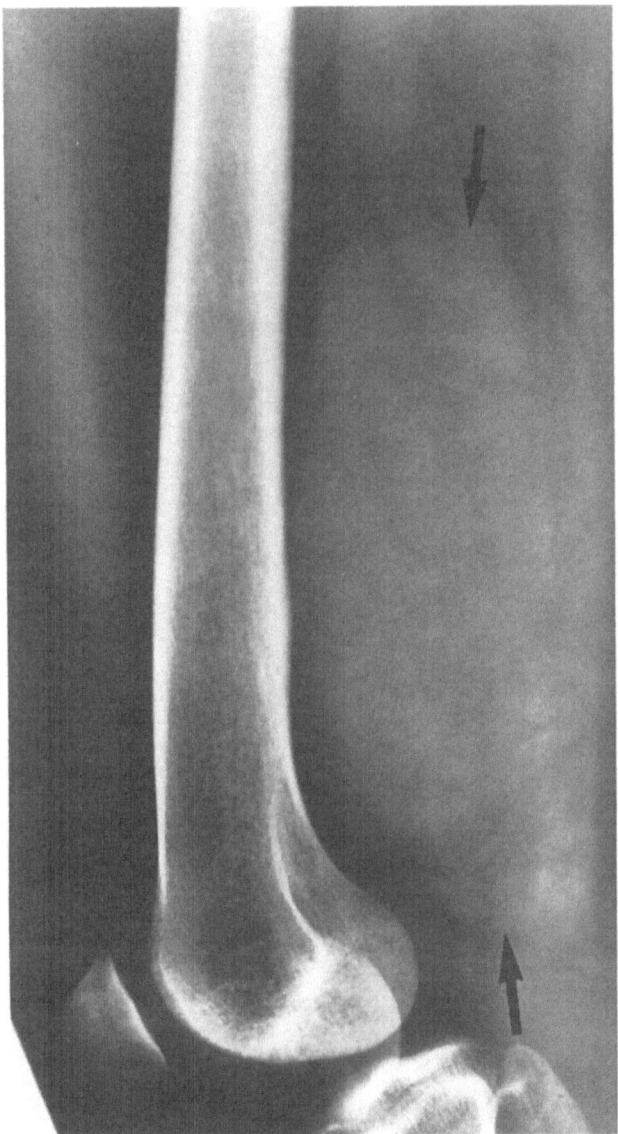

Fig. 1

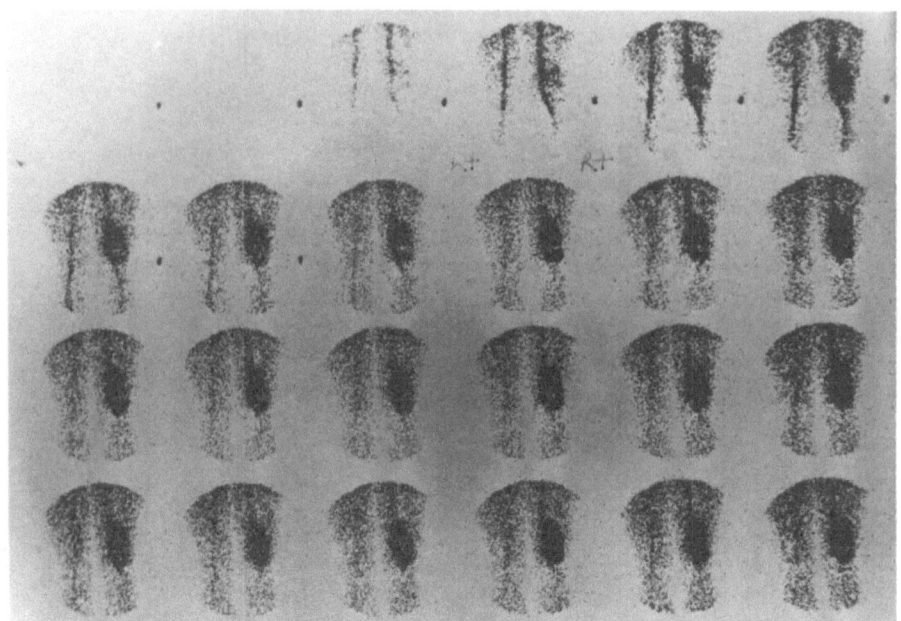

a

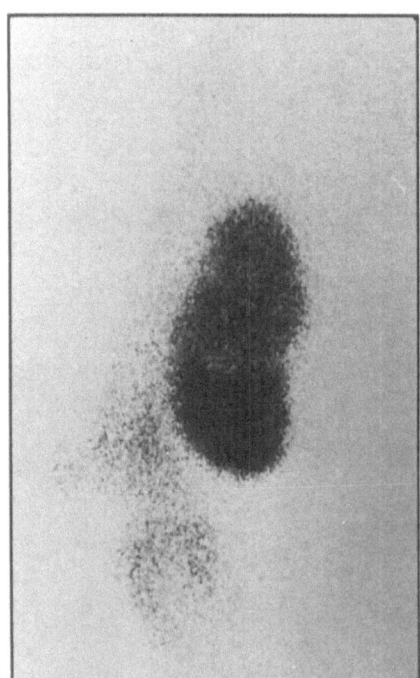

b

Fig. 2

Case 3

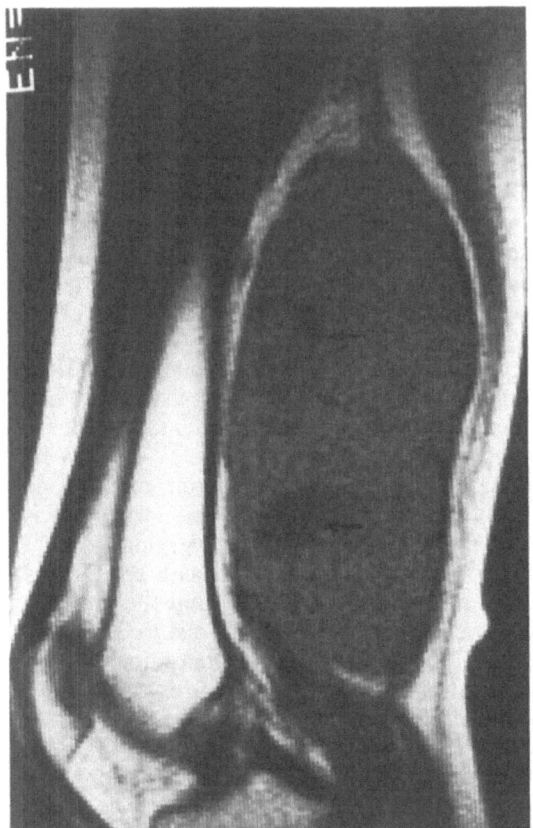

Fig. 3

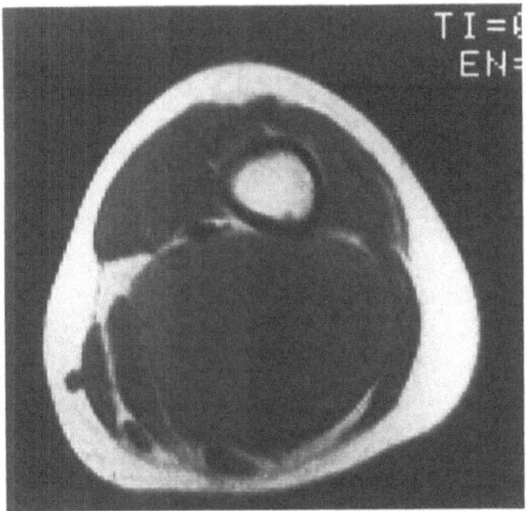

Fig. 4

Case 4

A 34-year-old female had a 4-month history of increasing knee pain and a rapidly developing mass in the anterior lateral leg just inferior to her knee. On physical examination there was a large tender firm mass just below the knee and anterior to the fibula. There was increased warmth to the touch.

The AP radiograph (case 4, Fig. 1) reveals a geographic lesion in the lateral proximal tibia with a narrow transition zone, complete destruction of the cortex and the suggestion of a soft tissue component.

This is clearly an aggressive lesion from both a radiographic and a clinical point of view, and further diagnostic work-up should include at least scintigraphy and CT.

Bone scintigraphy (case 4, Fig. 2) reveals increased uptake in the proximal tibia which extends beyond the area seen on the plain film, including a soft tissue (extraosseous) component. There is also increased uptake in the distal femur, probably secondary to disuse osteoporosis. No other abnormalities are seen.

The CT examination (case 4, Fig. 3a,b) clearly shows destruction of the bone and a large soft tissue component without a reactive rim of bone. The tumor is quite inhomogeneous (case 4, Fig. 3b) with attenuation values varying from 31 to 56 HU before intravenous infusion of contrast medium and with some areas being markedly enhanced during infusion. The inhomogeneity and the presence of areas showing no enhancement on intravenous infusion of contrast medium suggest areas of necrosis within the tumor. There is extension of the tumor through the intraosseous membrane. The exact relationship between the neurovascular bundle posteriorly and the lesion cannot be identified on the CT scan.

A digital angiogram was carried out. In the lateral projection (case 4, Fig. 4) there was no evidence of displacement of the popliteal artery or posterior tibial or anterior tibial artery.

To delineate possible intra-articular extension of the tumor, MRI was performed. In the sagittal sections (case 4, Fig. 5) the subchondral bone can be seen to be intact and there is no evidence of intra-articular extension.

The radiologic chest examination was normal.

Evaluation of the clinical and radiographic findings suggests an aggressive lesion consistent with either an aggressive benign process, possibly a giant cell tumor, or a malignant tumor.

An incisional biopsy revealed a giant cell tumor of the bone and the patient was treated with a resection of the proximal tibia and a reconstruction allograft.

Surgical stage: 3.

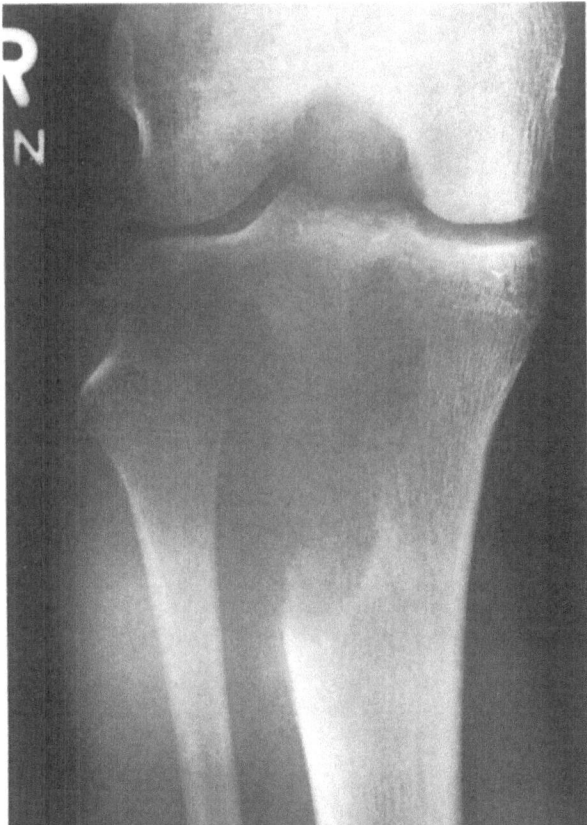

Fig. 1

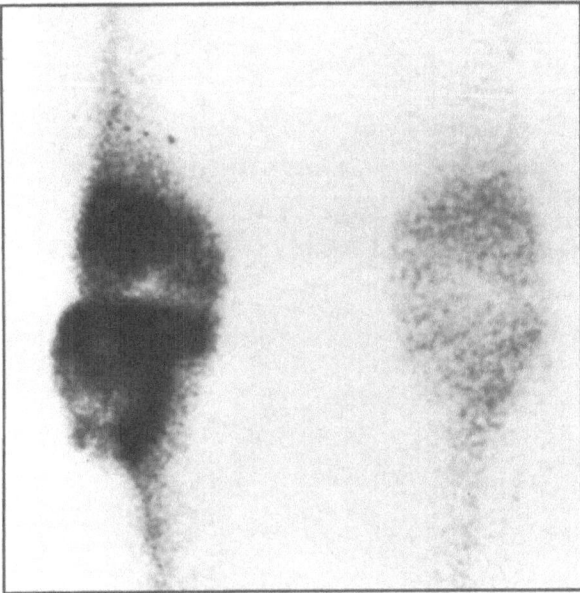

Fig. 2

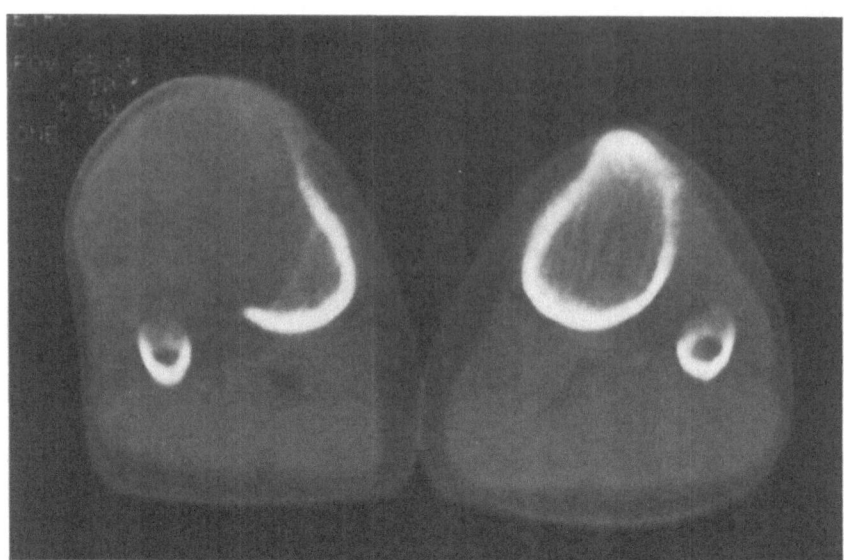

a

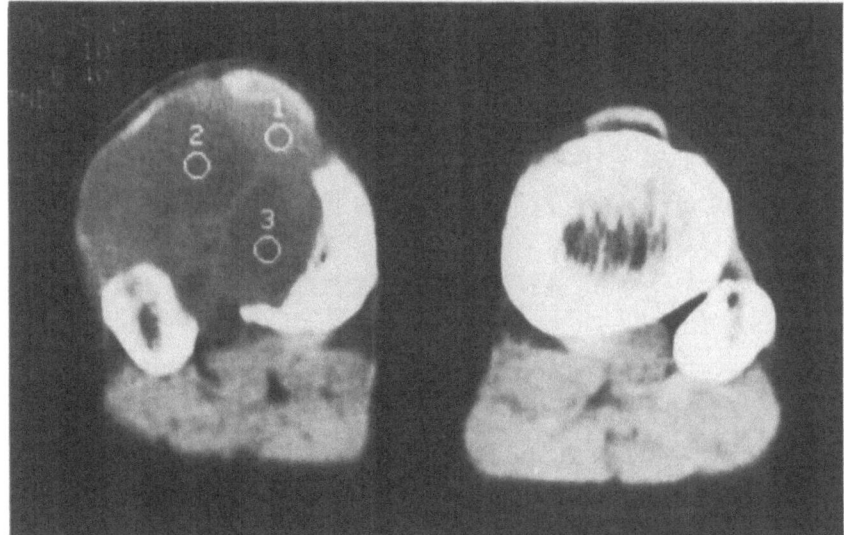

b

Fig. 3

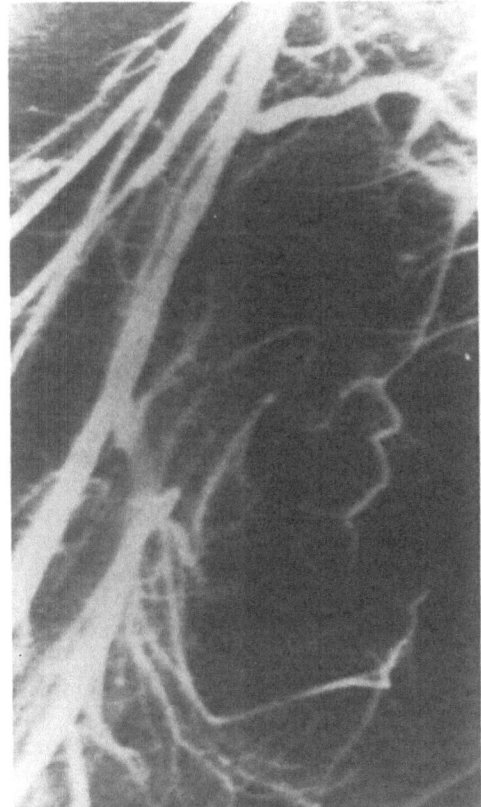

Fig. 4

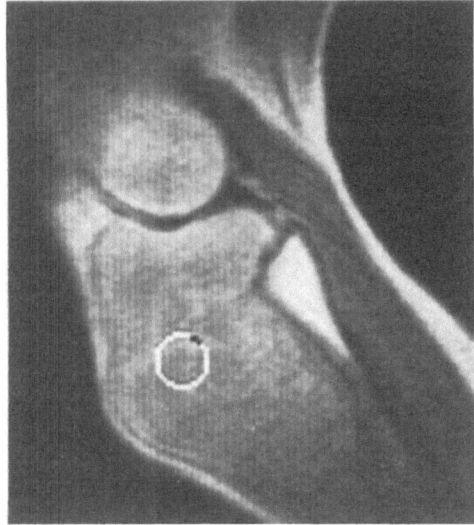

Fig. 5

Case 5

A 50-year-old male had a 6-month history of an aching pain in the thigh, progressively getting worse. The symptoms were not related to activity and occasionally awakened him at night. The patient's past medical history was unremarkable. He had no evidence of infection. On physical examination there was no palpable mass in the thigh and the leg functioned normally.

On the AP plain radiograph (case 5, Fig. 1) there is evidence of deformity of the cortex in the subtrochanter area, producing the so-called expanded appearance. This expansion of a bone suggests that the lesion has eroded the endosteal surface but is growing so slowly that the periosteum is able to make a new cortex. There is loss of the intermedullary trabecular pattern distal to the base of the femoral neck. Radiographically this is an active lesion, and given the patient's age and symptoms it should be regarded as potentially malignant.

Scintigraphy (case 5, Fig. 2) reveals increased activity from the distal femoral shaft up into the femoral neck. No other areas of increased activity were found.

The CT examination (case 5, Fig. 3) reveals generally increased attenuation values within the medullary canal, with dispersed areas of calcification. There is no evidence of cortical destruction or extraosseous mass.

The radiologic chest examination was normal.

The clinical setting and radiologic findings are consistent with an active tumor, potentially fibrous dysplasia, Paget's disease, or low-grade intraosseous chondrosarcoma.

An incisional biopsy was done through the greater trochanter so that minimal tissue was contaminated, and the diagnosis of low-grade chondrosarcoma was made. The patient was treated with a resection of the entire femur. The tumor was found to be totally intraosseous.

Surgical stage: IA.

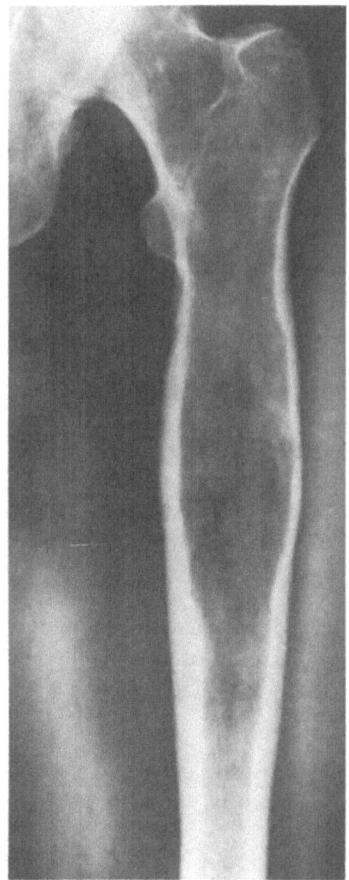

Fig. 1

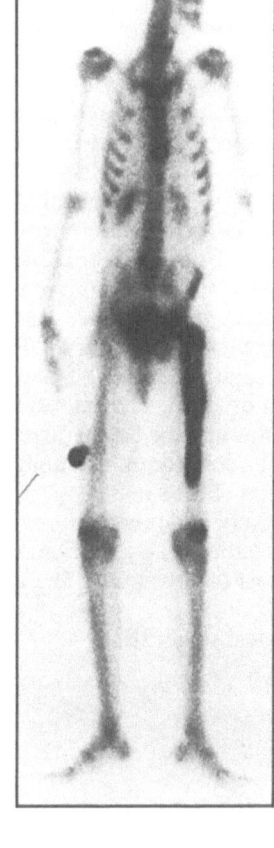
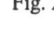

Fig. 2

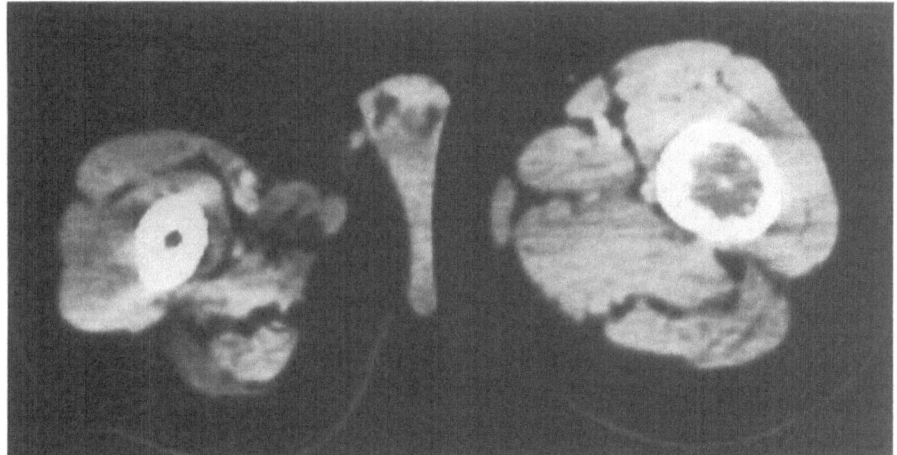

Fig. 3

Case 6

A 50-year-old female presented with low back pain for 1 year. Her neurologic examination was normal but on rectal examination a tender mass was felt attached to the sacrum.

A lateral radiograph (case 6, Fig. 1) shows destruction of the distal sacrum and coccyx and a soft tissue mass attached to the distal end of the preserved bone (arrows).

The lateral projection of the scintigraphy (case 6, Fig. 2) shows no increased activity. In spite of the negative scintigraphy results the radiograph indicates an aggressive lesion and the clinical setting is typical of a chordoma.

At the CT examination (case 6, Fig. 3) a central mass involving the coccyx and distal sacrum is seen protruding both anteriorly into the pelvis and posteriorly. In the center of the lesion there is an area of calcification.

The sagittal section of the MRI examination (case 6, Fig. 4) better delineates the tumor. Proximal extension into S3 is obvious, as is the layer of fat between the tumor and the bowel (arrow). Our experience has been that MRI is particularly useful in delineating the anatomic extent of lesions which involve the soft tissue and bone of the spine.

The radiologic chest examination was normal.

This patient had an incisional biopsy which confirmed the clinical and radiologic diagnosis of chordoma. She then had a wide surgical resection of her distal spine from S2 distal.

Surgical stage: IB.

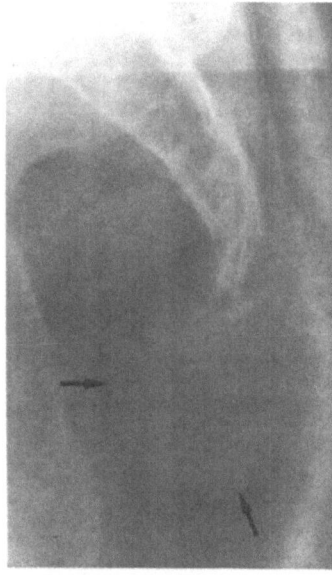

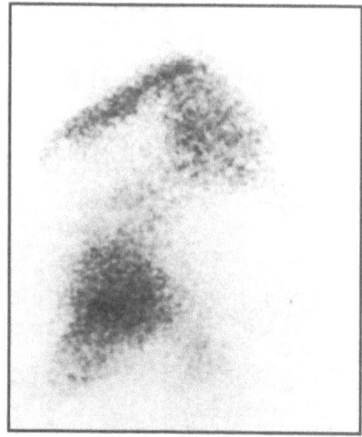

Fig. 1   Fig. 2

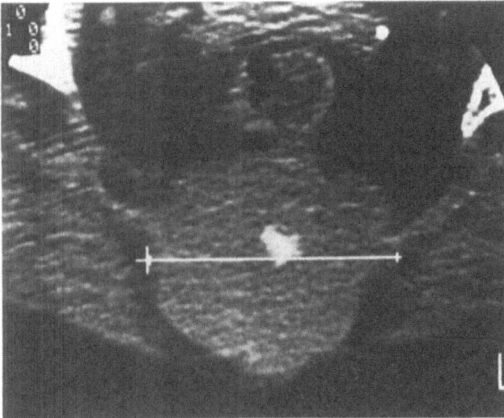

Fig. 3

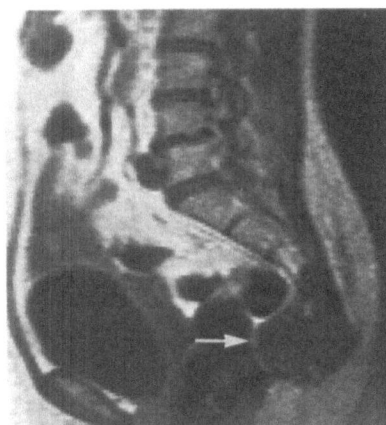

Fig. 4

Case 7

An 18-year-old female had an injury at work, and therefore had a radiograph taken of her distal femur. She was asymptomatic.

On the AP radiograph (case 7, Fig. 1a) there is an irregular and inhomogeneous dense area within the medial metaphysis extending into the epiphysis. The bone is otherwise normal. On an oblique view (case 7, Fig. 1b) it is apparent that as well as the dense area being inhomogeneous, there is a diffuse border between it and the normal bone, suggesting an active lesion.

It was felt that further investigation was indicated despite the patient's lack of symptoms. This was particularly true because the patient was a teenager with a bone-forming lesion that could not be specifically identified as a recognizable benign process.

Scintigraphy was performed (case 7, Fig. 2), which revealed increased uptake extending slightly farther than the dense area seen on the plain film. This suggests an active or aggressive bone-forming process, and further evaluation with CT is indicated.

At the CT examination (case 7, Fig. 3) the area of increased bone formation is seen to be situated in the medial femoral condyle, to be confined to the bone, and to involve the cortex and medullary canal. As the plain film suggested, the new bone formation appears inhomogeneous.

The radiologic chest examination was normal.

Because the patient was a teenager with a bone-forming lesion in the distal femur, and despite the fact that she had a normal serum alkaline phosphatase level, osteogenic sarcoma could not be excluded, and therefore, a biopsy was indicated. It revealed a high-grade osteogenic sarcoma. The patient was treated with a limb-salvage resection and chemotherapy.

Surgical stage: IIA.

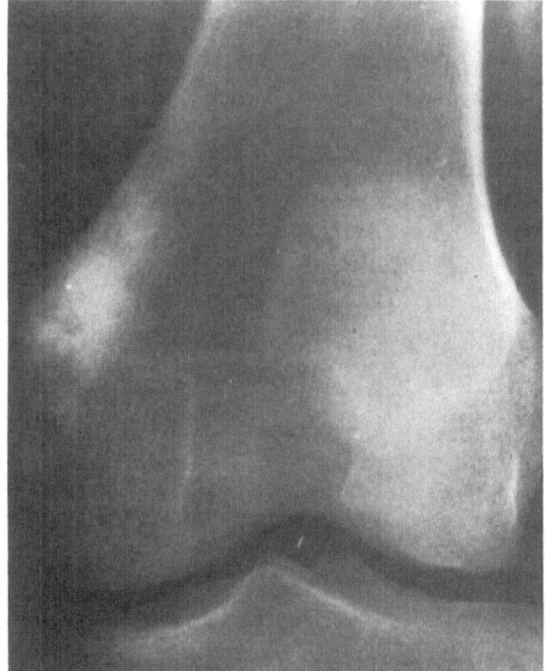

a

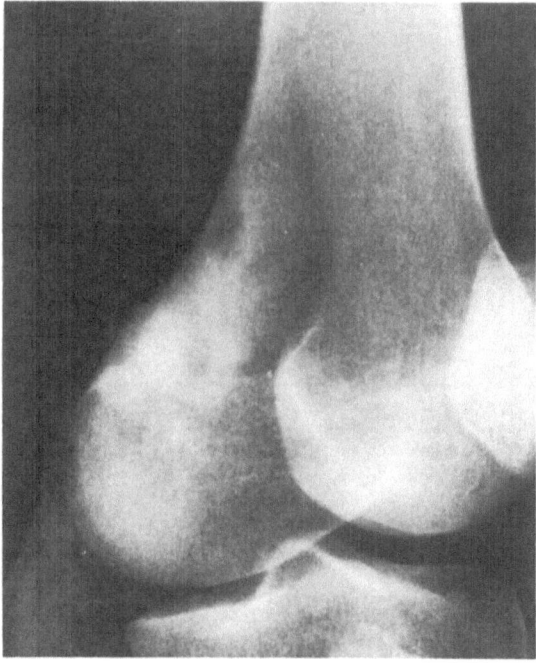

b

Fig. 1

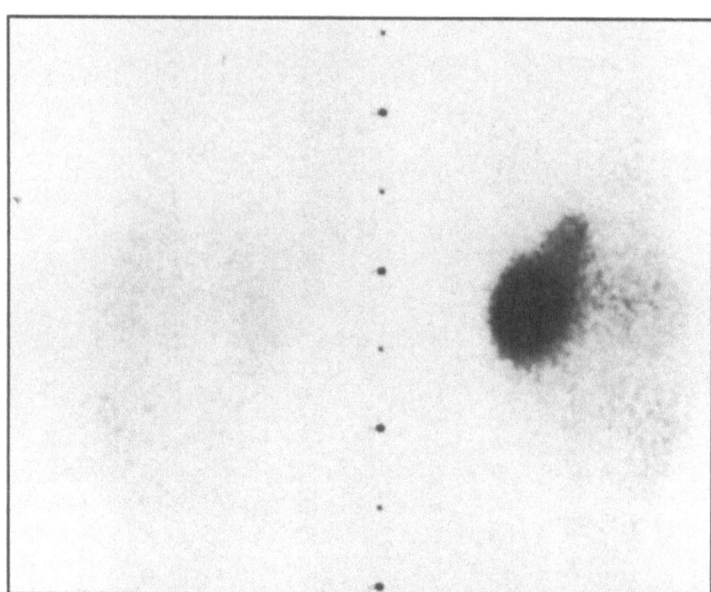
Fig. 2

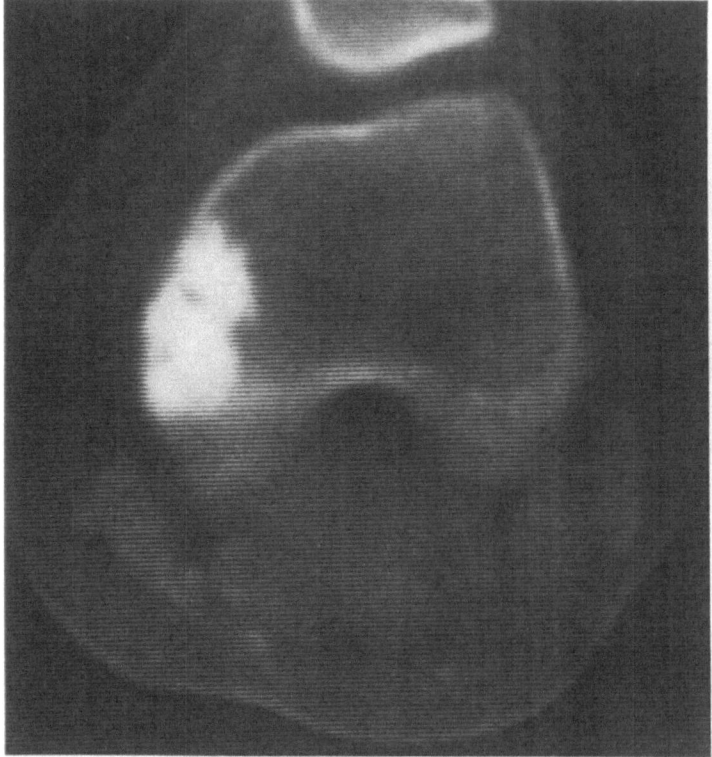
Fig. 3

Case 8

A 24-year-old female presented with an enlarging mass in the left lower quadrant of the abdomen associated with minimal symptoms. On physical examination there was a hard mass in her left lower quadrant which was fixed to the pelvis. The patient was able to ambulate without difficulty and the neurovascular examination of the left lower extremity was normal.

The AP radiograph of the pelvis (case 8, Fig. 1) shows a soft tissue density filling the left lower quadrant and iliac fossa, with evidence of ossification and calcification within the lesion. The underlying bone appears grossly normal.

An AP spot view from the scintigraphy (case 8, Fig. 2) shows no activity within the lesion itself, but there is decreased activity in the posterior ilium compared with the contralateral side (arrow). There were no other areas of increased activity on the bone scan.

A CT examination of the pelvis and lower abdomen and spine was done (case 8, Figs. 3a,b). In the true pelvis the tumor is seen to fill the left lower quadrant, displacing the bladder and the right common iliac artery to the right side. The lesion is immediately adjacent to the ilium. Most of the tumor has a low attenuation value with scattered calcifications.

The lesion extends proximally (case 8, Fig. 3b) in the retroperitoneum above the iliac crest, crosses the midline and is immediately adjacent to the vertebral bodies. Bone windows (case 8, Fig. 4) reveal destruction of the inner cortex of the ilium and calcification within the lesion.

An arteriogram (case 8, Fig. 5a) shows displacement of the distal aorta, common iliac, and external iliac arteries. In the late venous phase (case 8, Fig. 5b) the compressed iliac vein is seen. During or after angiographic procedures, particularly for pelvic lesions, the contrast medium injected should also be used for a survey of the kidneys and ureters (case 8, Fig. 6). As in the present case, the displacement of the ureter is often obvious.

The frontal MRI sections (case 8, Figs. 7a,b) reveal the extent of the tumor in the pelvis, particularly its relationship to the common iliac artery, which is displaced medially (case 8, Fig. 7a). Note the normal uterus compressing the bladder. More posterior frontal sections show the relationship to both the iliac wing and the lower spine (case 8, Fig. 7b).

Transaxial MRI sections also reveal the relationship between the lower vertebral column and the tumor (case 8, Fig. 8a) as well as the involvement of the iliac bone, and a skip lesion lateral to the iliac bone (case 8, Fig. 8b; arrow).

The plain chest radiograph and the chest CT showed no evidence of metastatic disease.

An incisional biopsy revealed a high-grade primary chondrosarcoma and the patient underwent preoperative chemotherapy and radiotherapy and then had an extended hemipelvectomy. A photograph of the cut section of the specimen through the ilium (case 8, Fig. 9) shows the relationship of the tumor to the ilium: it is intimately associated with the inner wall. As seen on the MRI, there is a skip lesion on the outer wall of the ilium.

Surgical stage: IIB.

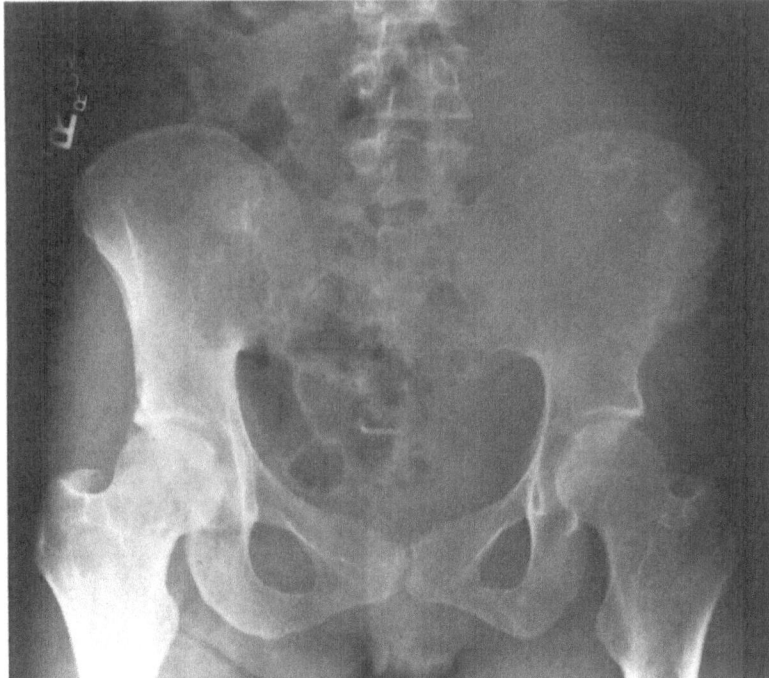

Fig. 1

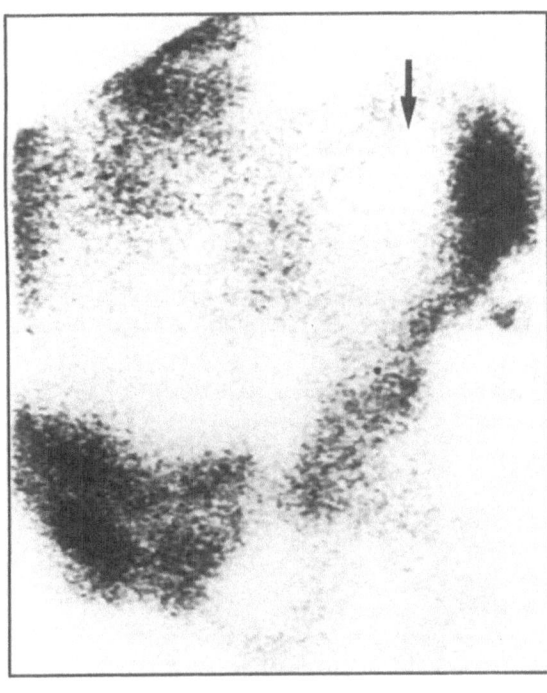

Fig. 2

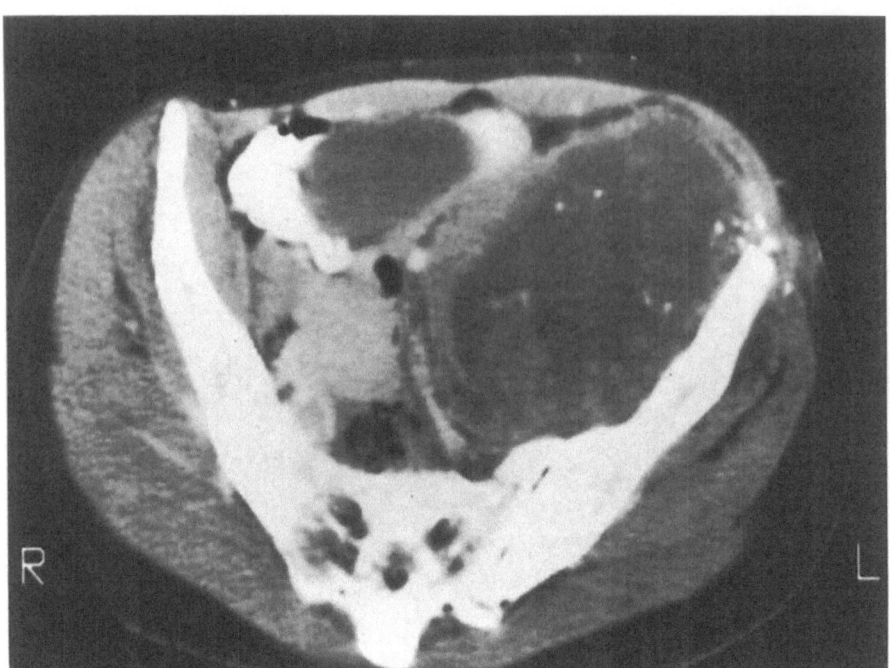

a

b

Fig. 3

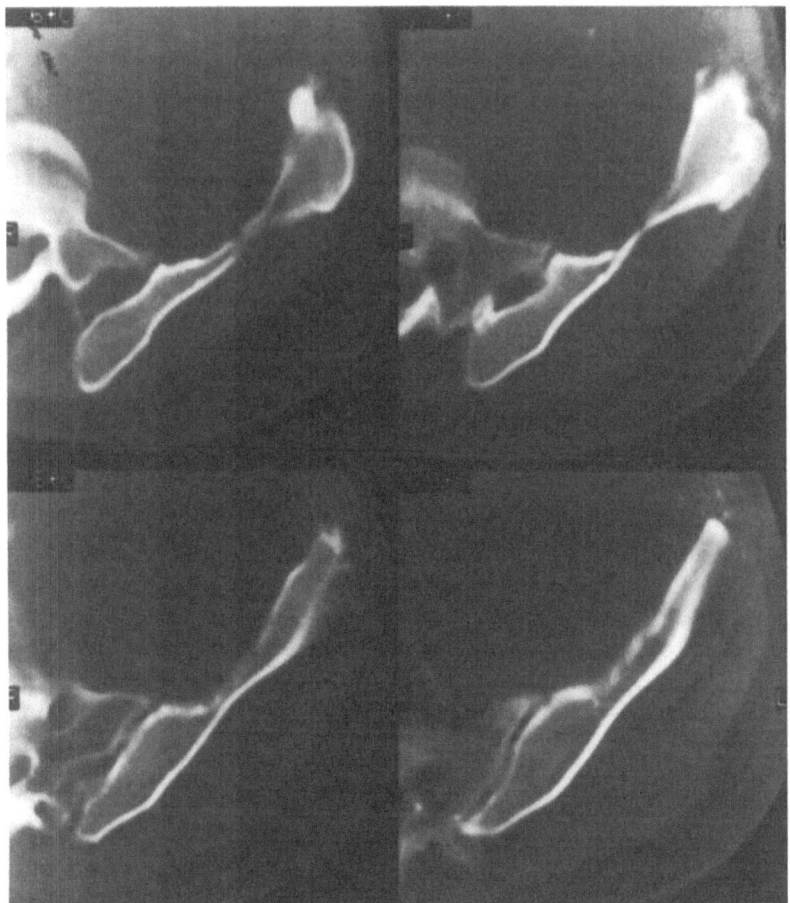

Fig. 4

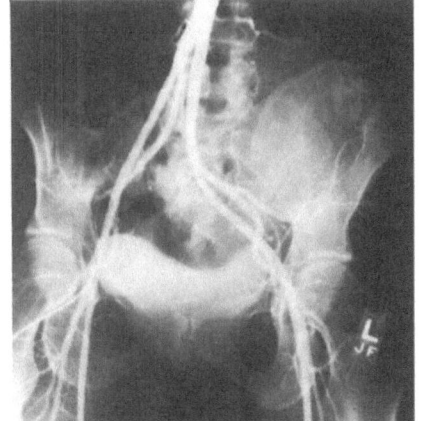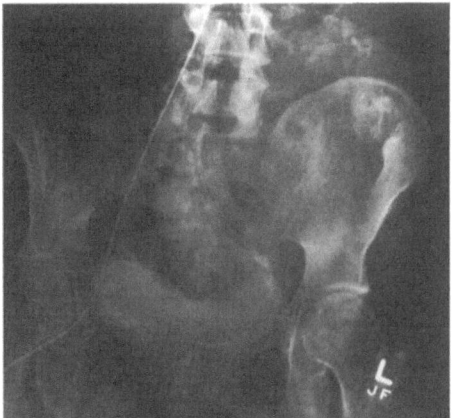

a   b

Fig. 5

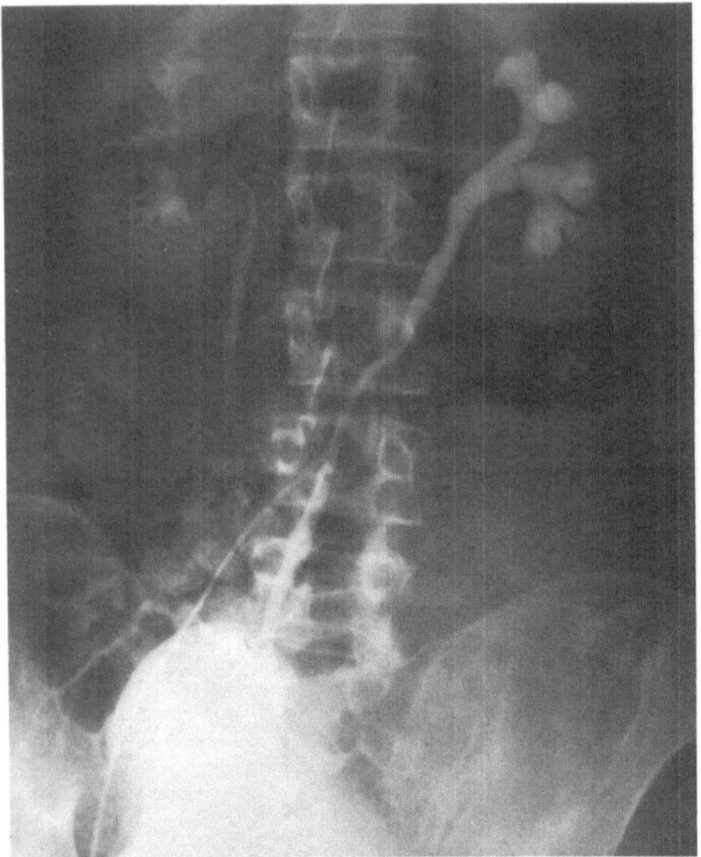

Fig. 6

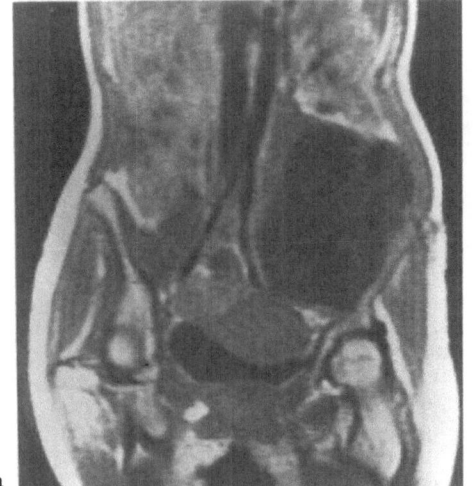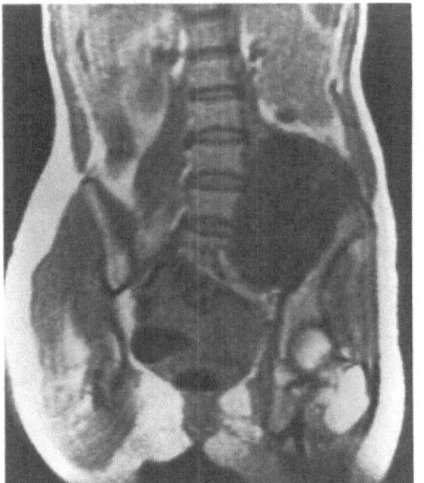

a   b

Fig. 7

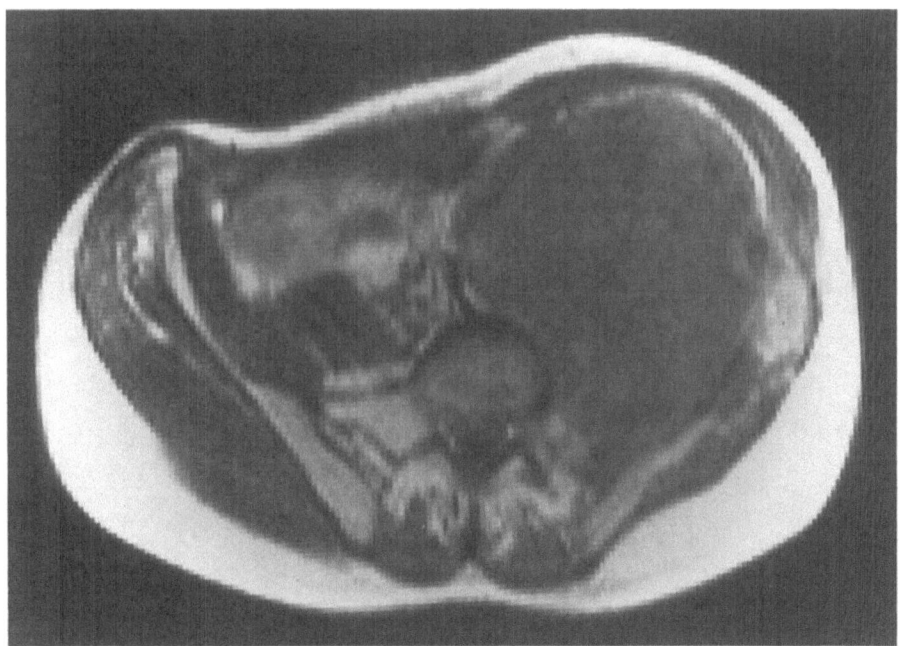

a

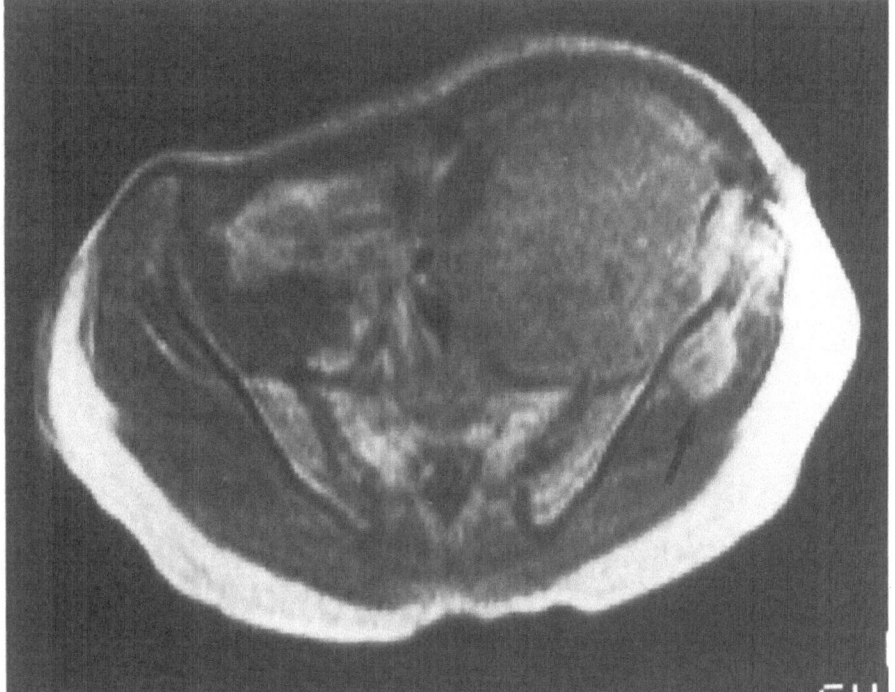

b

Fig. 8

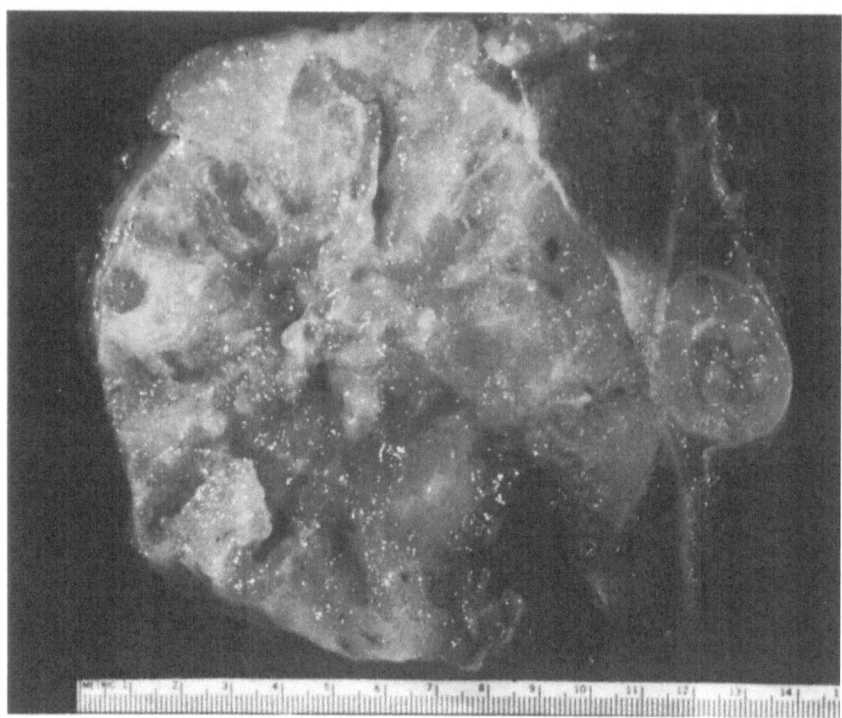

Fig. 9

Case 9

A 70-year-old male had an enlarging mass in the medial thigh for approximately 1 month. On physical examination there was a firm, minimally tender mass deep to the subcutaneous tissue in the area of the adductor canal. The distal vascular supply was normal as were the neurologic findings in the distal part of the extremity. The mass measured approximately 8 cm × 10 cm.

The plain radiograph (case 9, Fig. 1) suggests a soft tissue mass in the medial thigh without bone involvement. There are no calcifications within the lesion.

Soft tissue tumors in adults should be considered malignant until proved otherwise, and therefore further radiologic examination was indicated.

Scintigraphy (case 9, Fig. 2) reveals increased uptake within the lesion. There is a surgical margin between the tumor and the bone, indicated by the area of soft tissue with normal uptake between them.

The MRI (case 9, Fig. 3) shows a tumor in the medial anterior compartment of the thigh which appears to grow circumferentially around the neurovascular bundle. There is normal tissue between the bone and the tumor.

Because of the anatomic location of this lesion an arteriogram was obtained (case 9, Fig. 4). Not only is there evidence of atherosclerotic disease, but there is also a constriction of the femoral artery with tumor on each side, indicating that the artery is encased within the tumor.

The radiologic chest examination was normal.

The patient underwent a surgical resection, and the tumor was found to encase the neurovascular bundle circumferentially (case 7, Fig. 5). The histologic examination revealed a high-grade malignant fibrous histiocytoma.

Surgical stage: IIB.

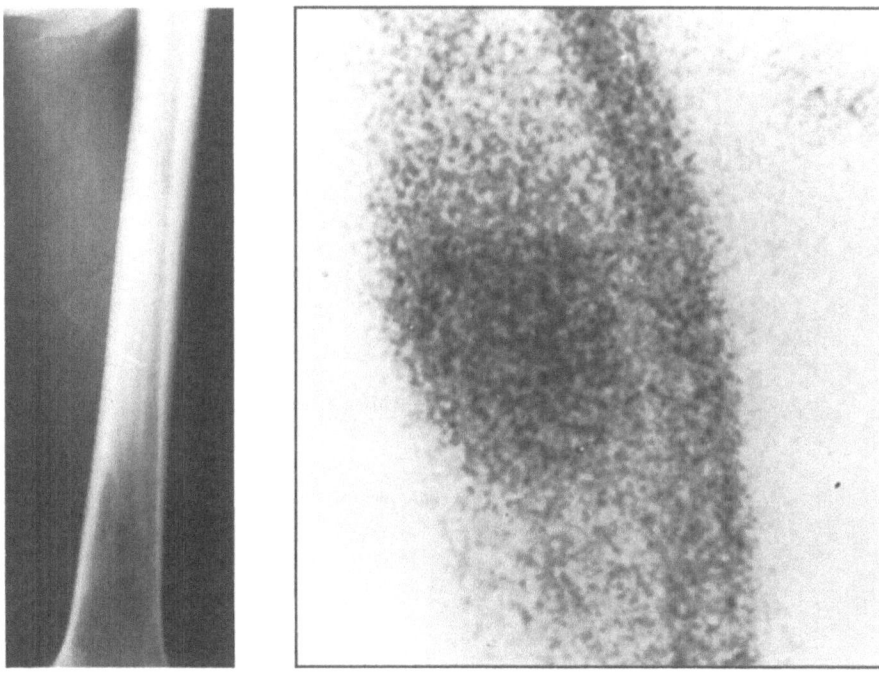

Fig. 1   Fig. 2

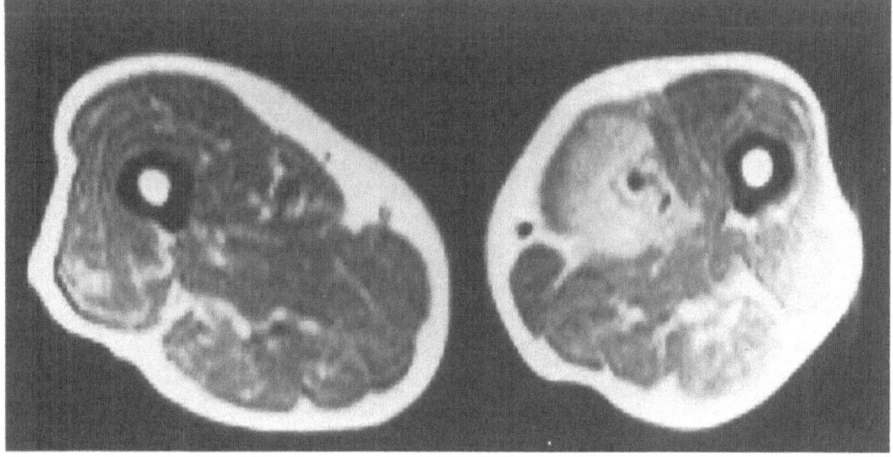

Fig. 3

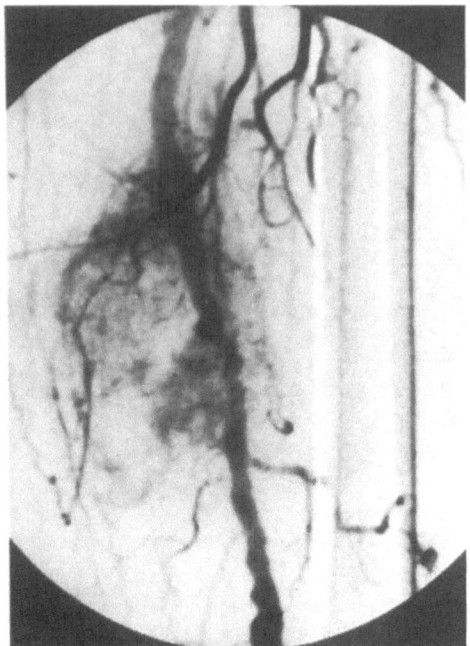

Fig. 4

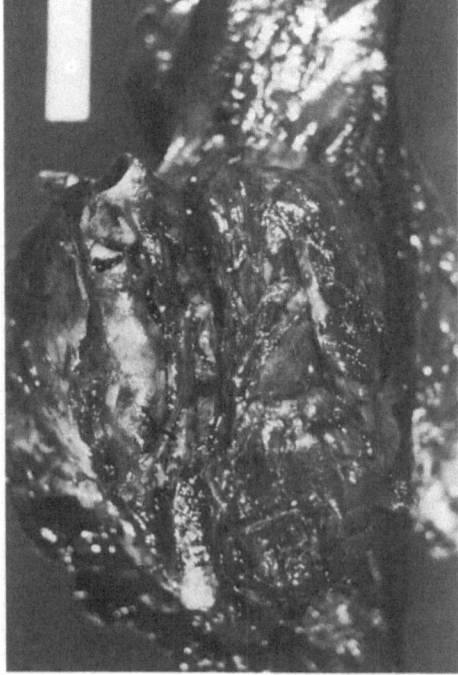

Fig. 5

Subject Index